"We know conventional medicine is not enough because the cancer comes back too often. Immersive Healing is an evidence-based treatment designed to heal the mind patterns that created illness in the first place"

Avinoam Lerner

"We cannot change the wind but we can adjust our Sails"
(Author unknown)

thank you sarah for helping me do just that.

Avinoam

Library of Congress Control Number: 2012919144

ISBN 978-1480079939
ISBN 1480079936

AvinoamLerner.com
Free@AvinoamLerner.com

Printed in North Charleston, SC

The
New Cancer Paradigm

Increase the Effectiveness of Your Medical
Treatment with Immersive Healing

By Avinoam Lerner

Cover by damonza.com

I dedicate this book to my wife Ruth.
She inspires me every day to be all that I can be.

About Avinoam Lerner

Avinoam Lerner is a holistic therapist and a certified hypnotherapist. He earned his degree in Holistic Health from the Reidman International College for Complementary and Integrative Medicine in Israel in 2000.

He is certified by the National Guild of Hypnotists (NGH) and the National Federation of Neuro Linguistic Programming (NLP) in the USA.

Since beginning to study ancient and modern healing practices in the Far East in 1992, Avinoam has developed his ability to help clients transform physical and emotional suffering into wellness and serenity.

In his private practice in Brookline, Massachusetts he helps those touched by chronic illness and cancer to heal from within.

He calls upon a wide spectrum of evidence-based holistic disciplines in his healing sessions and tailors them to fit individual client's need.

In 2006 he received a Letter of Commendation from the Mayor of Newton, Massachusetts for the support he had been providing to those with cancer, anxiety attacks and emotional turmoil.

In an article entitled "Therapist uses hypnosis as a weapon "(Jewish Advocate, 2012), Jason M. Rubin quoted Avinoam Lerner as saying: *"If we have a toxic message broadcast over and over in our minds, it becomes the truth we live by. And that truth makes us vulnerable to illness."*.....*"That idea is core to Avinoam Lerner's approach to healing."*

Acknowledgement

A special tribute to Stephen Parkhill, the author of *Answer Cancer – the Healing of a Nation* for developing and perfecting the practice of Hypnotic Regression to Cause for healing Cancer. His knowledge, insights and unmatched creativity are the foundation and inspiration for *Immersive Healing*.

Immersive Healing was also inspired by the invaluable work of Dr. Alfred Barrios who laid the foundation for the practice of Hypnotherapy as an Immunotherapeutic approach to healing cancer. In 1996 Dr. Barrios received the first annual Cancer Federation Award in Psychoneuroimmunology and nominated for the Norman Cousins Award in Mind-Body Health.

Foreword

Understanding the role and purpose of illness requires recognition of its primary message. Illness is a call for us to take action. It is a call for us to actively participate in our own healing. Illness highlights the necessity and inevitability of an existential shift to live more authentically, aligned with our sincere and relevant core values. Illness forces us to understand and face its meaning and purpose. It is a call to take action and to actively participate in the creation of our own lives.

There is much more to cancer than only what the doctors can see, measure or touch. Therefore, the journey toward healing and health must include more than *only* what happens during visits with your medical doctor. Illness affects us in many more ways than just *poor physical health*. Cancer affects every aspect of our physical and emotional life, so therefore, *healing requires more than only removing the physical cancer.*

The healing journey must include the acceptance of a meaning and purpose and the need to take action from within. Embracing your plan to heal requires answering this call to action. A *call to engage* the hidden meaning and purpose of the illness, *not ignore* it.

Illness highlights our inherent need to evolve on all levels. It propels us to look deep within and live more authentically.

Those who have healed view their illness as a "wake-up call" and an opportunity to re-prioritize life and claim a more authentic and spiritual approach to living (Choron, 1963, Grof and Halifax, 1978). For many, the suffering inherent in critical illness offers keys to unlock the doors of spiritual awareness and growth that have previously remained unopened. (Lerner, 1994).

It is only when we open these doors that we begin the process of real-life transformation. Reports of transformation are very common among patients who have had a remarkable recovery from a life-threatening illness such as cancer.

While studying terminally ill cancer patients who remitted "spontaneously" without any medical treatment, researchers discovered that many of these patients underwent a significant existential or spiritual shift in their thinking, their beliefs, and their way of being in the world. (Berland,) 1994, Hawley, 1989, Hirshberg and Barasch, 1995, Huebscher, 1992, Roud, 1985).

Among the factors contributing to healing, investigators reported changes of a "spiritual, religious, or existential nature", depending on the perspective both of the participants and the investigators. In almost all cases, the patients claimed a "profoundly altered sense of self which recognizes fulfillment and relatedness to something larger than the self."

When first diagnosed with cancer you may not care much for the above statements. Real-life transformation, a call to action, hidden purpose and meaning in illness, these may not make much sense at all. It is difficult in the beginning to understand that your illness can have a positive impact on your life. *Nevertheless, it's all true!*

The journey along the path to healing is not a fun or a pleasant trip. I do not pretend that there is anything pleasant about "being with" cancer or that healing cancer is an easy process. However, no matter how unpleasant this process is or how angry it makes you feel, do not deny your journey its purpose. At the very least, discovering the purpose and meaning of your illness will make this road less painful and less tiresome.

Knowledge of self-accumulated through experience cultivates wisdom. Wisdom will lead you out of the *dark forest of fear and the unknown* so you can see the way to a promising healing future, to a place where you can remember this truth: *While we may be with illness we are not our illness.*

Chapter 1

Introduction

"You have cancer!"

These are the most difficult words you may hear from your doctor. Either you or someone you know has cancer, and before hearing these three words was first a mother, father, son, daughter, friend or relative. The instant these words reached your ears, you became *a cancer patient*.

"Why Me?"

The answer to this troubling question cannot be found inside the tumor cells. You must look beyond viruses, organs, DNA and germs and into the realm of meaning and purpose to properly answer this question. You must transcend your opinion of illness and cancer as just an escalation of an uncontrollable group of malignant cells and look deeper within. Hidden within you is the right answer to the question... *Why Me?*

Your state of health is often synonymous with inner harmony. Illness is therefore a state of disharmony. This explains why it is such an uncomfortable and frightening experience for us to look within. We are afraid of what we might find. Nevertheless, it is the time to understand the answer to *Why Me* as a source for healing. Dreadful illness and dire situations beg the question, because the answer usually contains the missing piece to recovery.

Every cell in our body, all of our thoughts and all of our feelings are interrelated and inter-connected. When becoming afraid, the heart beat rate increases, blood pressure increases, sweating may occur and your thought process may be temporarily impaired. You could possibly go into cardiac arrest. My point is simple; *emotional messages result in physiological responses.*

The pattern of cause and effect sheds light on the mental patterns that contribute to our illness. It highlights our dominant thoughts, beliefs we practice, what works in our life and what does not. Discovering the hidden patterns will identify areas that need healing the most. In doing so, we identify the cause and what we need to; change, fix, repair, replace, update or totally abandon in our life. We reach to find the missing components to healing and recovery.

Why Me ... is your call to take action, to begin the journey of discovery. A journey to find hidden secrets within each of us, secrets waiting to be discovered. The secret to self-love, self-acceptance, courage, healing and compassion are all now within your reach.

This journey to discover these secrets was forced upon us because of illness. However, this journey is ultimately a freeing experience.

You can emerge from your journey *reborn, stronger, and happier and with a greater appreciation for the gift of life.*

The healing journey begins on the path of discovery where choices, decisions, and self-participation are required. This journey is not necessarily easy. It requires strength, courage and action. Many of my clients effectively mobilized all of their resources in order to face one of the most difficult challenges in their life.

You seek answers to the following questions:

- What can I do to improve my own recovery and healing?

- How can I heal faster, better and stronger?
- Are there ways I can supplement the doctor's treatment?
- How can I remain positive during my recovery?

I discuss these questions and many others in the hope that this book will make it very clear that trying to heal cancer solely by destroying tumors is only one part of your healing process.

Cancer cells and tumors are the manifestations of a deeper condition. Unfortunately, results show that far too often the cancer reappears if the systemic condition that nurtured the illness is not also healed.

Removing only the cancer tumor has brought dismal results for so many patients for so many years. The current mindset of cut, burn or poison the tumor has dominated cancer care for more than 60 years. You can remove the tumor, but unless you change the conditions that nurtured its creation in the first place, it can simply start again somewhere else in the body. I strongly support the argument and research that placing focus solely on the physical cancer remains a problem with the current approach to treatment.

The tumor can reappear very quickly. Studies of postoperative cancer patients show that when a tumor is surgically removed, growth signals associated with wound healing can sometimes be unleashed, triggering any remaining malignant cells to grow and develop into a new tumor.

The good news is that Immersive Healing will heal the Mind aspects that agitated and stressed the body's internal environment over many years, disrupted its proper functioning and produced the conditions where illness can thrive.

Immersive Healing lets you choose living and health over illness. Choosing living and health over illness means you must embrace healing and take action daily during your journey. To embrace healing requires the right integrative Mind and Body approach that will heal the root cause of the illness. In this book, I discuss a journey that allows you to reclaim your health using an approach that puts you in control of your own healing to reclaim control of your life.

You can improve your odds of success for recovery and health, with more options than you realize exist. This is why you must begin the journey by ignoring survival rates, remission rates, and other cancer statistics. *Those numbers need not apply to you.* Continue your journey ahead!

Chapter 2

The Current Paradigm for Medical Cancer Treatment

On Friday afternoon Dr. Philip West left the hospital for the weekend believing he would not see his patient, Mr. Wright, alive on Monday. Mr. Wright had lymphosarcoma, a generalized and advanced malignancy of the lymph nodes. Tumors the size of oranges already spread through his body; his vital organs were failing, and a full time oxygen mask was required to support his breathing. Mr. Wright's prognosis was a textbook case of the word *terminal.* His chances of recovery were so poor that Dr. West did not expect him to survive the night, let alone the weekend.

Even though he did not qualify to participate in the clinical research study because of his prognosis, Mr. Wright convinced Dr. West to treat him with Krebiozen. By all accounts of what Mr. Wright read, there was *not one iota of doubt in his Mind,* the new treatment was going to work. Wright felt positive and convinced that Krebiozen would be his answer and heal him.

On the other hand, Dr. West held the opinion that Krebiozen would not work for Mr. Wright. Furthermore, he did not want to include a patient destined not to survive and thus skew the statistical results of the clinical study. However, after much convincing, Dr. West yielded to Mr. Wright's persuasive appeal. He agreed to administer an initial dose of the new drug before he left on Friday afternoon. Dr. West thought denying Mr. Wright's personal plea would have been too cruel, especially since he felt so optimistic. Against Dr. West's better professional judgment, he injected Mr. Wright with a single dose of the new drug Krebiozen. He did so, but only outside the scope of the official clinical research and not as part of the study.

Dr. West returned to the hospital Monday morning to discover that Mr. Wright survived the weekend. Not only did he survive, but Dr. West also found an alert, bright-eyed, energetic patient breathing on his own and out of bed. In amazement, the doctor discovered the tumors were half their original size since Friday. The doctor was totally in awe!

"I left him febrile, gasping for air and bedridden, and now here he is walking around the ward, chatting happily with the nurses and spreading his message of good cheer to anyone who would listen" reported Dr. West.

He was filled with joy in the belief that *a cure for cancer finally arrived.* Immediately, he visited the other clinical trial patients to observe their improvement. Imagine his enthusiasm thinking of the millions of people this new treatment would help.

However, he soon discovered that none of the other clinical trial patients showed any improvement whatsoever. Mr. Wright was the only patient with such a remarkable improvement. The tumor masses melted like *snowballs on a hot stove.* In only a few days, the tumors shrank to half their original size. He had no other treatment, just one single dose injection.

Within ten days he was cancer free, discharged from the hospital and sent home. He was breathing normally, active, and free of pain.

Dr. West had no logical explanation. What was it about the drug, or Mr. Wright, that caused his extraordinary recovery? No one else experienced any benefit. What contributed to Wright's phenomenal recovery?

Two months later, reports from the clinical trial study were released. Krebiozen proved ineffective for cancer treatment. All of its promising benefits were unproven. Shortly after Mr. Wright read the clinical report news, he was re-admitted to the hospital. He was again ill, depressed, weak, suffering a relapse.

Thinking the circumstance extreme enough to justify extraordinary measures, Dr. West told his patient that he was giving him a new, refined, double-strength dose of Krebiozen. Instead, West injected him with sterile water.

Wright's results were even more remarkable than the first time. Once again, the tumor masses melted, chest fluid vanished, and he became fully mobile and returned home. Remaining symptom-free for more than two months, it became clear that the patient's belief *alone* produced his recovery. Once again, the size of the tumors reduced, his strength restored, and Mr. Wright was again discharged and sent home as "the picture of health".

The final announcement from the American Medical Association (AMA) and the US Food and Drug Administration (FDA) appeared in the news *'Nationwide Clinical Test Trial Results Prove Krebiozen to be Powerless in the Treatment of Cancer.'*

As the reported results of clinical trials for Krebiozen studies became increasingly dismal and upon the news, Mr. Wright's faith sadly disappeared. After the first two months of astonishing perfect health, he relapsed to his original state. His belief was now gone, and his last hope for survival vanished. He relapsed to his original terminal condition, and this time did not survive the weekend. Mr. Wright died within a few days.

Dr. West logically concluded that Mr. Wright's recovery was a result of his powerful strong belief that Krebiozen would work for him. His *belief and hope* caused the tumors to shrink and disappear even in his hopeless, terminal condition. When his confidence and belief in the drug ended, so did his body's ability to resist the disease.

The first time I read this story was in Dr. Bernie Siegel's book *Love, Medicine & Miracles* (1986). Mr. Wright's story inspired me in many ways. This story literally caused a shift in the focus of my practice from general healing to the healing of cancer.

Mr. Wright was able to overcome the illness, not once but twice. The power of the Mind combined with the role of strong belief to heal and influence health is indisputable. As Dr. West assessed, once his confidence and belief ended, so did his resistance to the disease as well. In other words, his Immune System shut down when he no longer believed in the capacity of the treatment to heal.

Mr. Wright's experience of the Minds immense power to influence healing is not new. For centuries, many cultures around the world have acknowledged Mind over body as one of the most effective forms of healing.

Our Cancer Paradigm

We are fortunate to live in a time when the wonders of modern Medicine continue to evolve. New drugs, experimental treatments, new technology for early diagnosis, are results of extraordinary research from dedicated scientists and doctors.

The death rate from 2001 to 2007, for all cancers decreased by 1.9% each year in men and 1.5% per year from 2002 to 2007 in women. Compared with the peak rates in 1990 for men and 1991 for women -- the cancer death rate for all sites combined in 2007 was 22.2% lower in men and 13.9% lower in women. (American Cancer Society, Inc. ©2010)

This is great news, but statistics do not heal cancer. Statistics bring little or no comfort when battling cancer. The question is not *what are the odds of recovery for the world population,* but *what are my odds* of recovery *and how can I improve them?*

The current Paradigm consists of the conventional medical treatment, and the mindset presented by your doctors. Mainstream (allopathic) cancer treatments include surgery, chemotherapy, radiation and biotherapy. These treatments work within the scope of *only the physical dimension.*

Surgery

Surgery is usually the first course of action since it is clean, direct and offers the best chance of a cure. It aims to cut away all the tumor cells and as few of the healthy cells as possible. The hope, of course, is to minimize the chances that any malignant cells remain in the body, and the affected organs and related body systems will again function normal. Prognosis is best if diagnosed early, is localized, and has a low tendency to spread. Surgery may not be useful in certain types of cancers, especially blood cancers.

Chemotherapy

Chemotherapy aims to halt and reverse the uncontrolled growth of cells, using drugs. Chemotherapy is usually administered as a follow-up to surgery. On occasion, it is given before surgery in an attempt to reduce the size of the tumor. Chemotherapy carries a wide margin of error because, beyond a certain point, the therapeutic drugs cannot distinguish between healthy and cancerous cells. Your medical doctors will always require careful monitoring during this treatment.
Chemotherapy also has an adverse impact on the bone marrow, hair, skin, digestive tract and the Immune System,

leading to side effects such as fatigue, nausea, poor appetite, metallic taste, infections, bruising, bleeding, anemia and hair loss to name a few.

Recent technological advances have begun to allow doctors to target tumor cells more accurately.

Better genetic knowledge, more sensitive diagnostics, tailored drug formulations and calibrated dosages zero in on the individual tumor cells, to maximize the therapeutic effect and reduce the side effects.

Radiation

Radiation aims to thwart uncontrolled cell growth using gamma rays at approximately 10,000 times the intensity of normal X-rays.

It allows for targeted and controlled interventions that are most effective when the cancer is localized. Besides having similar side effects as chemotherapy, radiation produces a severe burning of surface and internal tissues. This can be very painful.

Biotherapy

Biotherapy is an emerging science, involving new techniques and approaches that introduce bio-chemicals such as antibodies, interferons and interleukins into the bloodstream.

These bio-chemicals stimulate the Immune System's own anti-cancer properties and encourage the self-repair of damaged genes.

Research and clinical trials are currently under way, and while the results are promising they are not yet conclusive.

Treatment Steps

Surgery is usually the first recourse. If surgery is successful and the tumor does not recur, the patient is classified as 'in remission' and is monitored regularly through blood tests, scans, etc.

A patient remaining in remission for five years is considered to be *recovered* by medical convention. A longer the period of remission usually means a lower risk of recurrence. For example, someone in remission for five years has the same probability of getting cancer as anyone else that has never had cancer.

Yet with all these variables and options, cancer treatment is still a hit-or-miss strategy. The Oncologist's skill is to determine the appropriate treatment methods, drugs and dosages for each type of cancer for each individual. Patients respond differently (or do not respond) to a specific regimen of treatment.

If the tumor completely disappears, shrinks or stops growing, the treatment is kept in *'maintenance' mode* to contain the tumor and keep it from spreading to other parts of the body. However, if the tumor continues to grow and spreads, then surgery may be repeated, and the chemotherapy or radiation treatments reapplied, often more aggressively. This process can take weeks and months, sometimes even years.

After trying all possible treatment combinations, if the tumor does not respond, then aggressive interventions may be discontinued and the focus then shifts to keeping the patient functional, comfortable and free of pain for the duration. Medical care provided by physicians, nurses and social workers that specialize in the relief of the pain symptoms and stress, is referred to as *palliative care.*

Why We Need a New Paradigm

The current cancer Paradigm places the focus only on the physical cancer, the tumor, and disease. We mistakenly provide our body to be treated as if it were only a pile of material to be removed, shifted around, and managed. The "state of disease" is brewing inside and can manifest itself in more ways than just the physical cancer.

Mind over Body

Although I am encouraged by the renewed emphasis on *emotional well-being*, I am also frustrated to discover its importance reduced to overly simple and trite views of *"just think positive"* or *"stress" management.* It represents so much more!

Positive thinking is clearly important, but positive thinking by itself is simply not enough to achieve healing. The expectation of preserving a calm Mind and positive mental attitude is overwhelming. It clearly sets us up for failure since we already feel helpless and overwhelmed facing the challenges of cancer.

Leading doctors agree to the importance of lowering stress levels, thinking positive and preserving hope and belief in treating cancer. Today, even a skeptic would agree there is strong evidence pointing to the power and ability of the Mind to change the physical body.

It is wonderful to see the importance of *emotional health* being recognized and encouraged as a contributing factor to healing. It helps to increase the chances of survival and quality of life. The problem is, "Mind over body" still focuses only on the results within the physical body. Mr. Wright's belief in the drug was a belief in a physical change, and thus unsustainable over time.

According to the Psychologist Dr.Klopfer who studied Mr. Wright's case, his recoveries were not sustainable because they were "not reinforced by the deep-rooted personality center. That would have counteracted the devastating effect of disappointing news about the drug's failure to cure cancer. His belief in the drug allowed for his extraordinary recovery, but it is important to note that his recovery was totally dependent on his perception and belief about Krebiozen."

Mr. Wright received an injection of sterile water instead of the real miracle drug, yet his Mind made the "drug" effective because his belief in the power of the drug to heal was complete. But it failed to sustain his health when the drug proved ineffective, because Mr. Wright did not have the same absolute belief in his own resources to heal and remain healthy.

What would have happened if Mr. Wright's Mind had resisted the news sources that told him, his treatment completely failed? What if Mr. Wright *believed* *i*n his recovery regardless of reports about the experimental clinical trials' statistics and resulting failed treatment?

It is possible for us to develop a Mind resistant to harmful external influence. Just as the body can be resistant to disease agents the Mind can be resistant to negative influences. In fact, they go hand and hand. The Mind and the body are not isolated and disconnected.

Incorporating the *Mind over body thinking* and *Mind-Body practices* into a cancer-fighting regiment is extremely useful, *but it still misses the point.* Mind over body alone still focuses on the recovery of the body. It still holds the body as the sole carrier of the disease.

The New Cancer Paradigm

As long as the cancer treatment focuses only on the body, we cannot expect to completely heal, not until the Mind is also healed. If the only object to be healed is the physical body, then only a partial and incomplete healing will take place. The missing piece is to heal not only the body, but also the Mind, the body's inseparable counterpart. We can only "partially" heal the body, unless we also heal the Mind! Healing one without healing the other does not complete the process or journey.

In the current Paradigm of thinking, cancer is a disease and our goal is recovery. In the new cancer Paradigm, cancer is an illness and the goal is to heal. You may think there is no difference, but as subtle as it may seem, these are two distinct perspectives of viewing cancer.

Disease

Disease is defined as "a disorder or incorrectly functioning organ, part, structure, or system of the body resulting from the effect of genetic or developmental errors, infection, poisons, nutritional deficiency or imbalance, toxicity, or unfavorable environmental factors, sickness, ailment." Cancer is looked upon as a structural and purely physical entity. It is viewed by the medical community as a physical condition that must be specifically targeted for treatment.

Yes, of course, the actual cancer cells must be treated! That is a given! But illness has a more holistic and less strict definition: *"unhealthy condition, poor health, indisposition, sickness."* Although there is a physical target, often an exceptionally clear one, the advantage of thinking of cancer as an illness, rather than disease, is its implication of something more than just the visible tumor.

It may be difficult to think of the cancer as anything bigger than the tumor, but a more complete and holistic view allows us to reach more potential sources, and therefore, more probable solutions.

Recovery and Healing

What is the difference between recovery and healing?

According to the on-line dictionary, to recover means to:

1. Get back or regain (*something lost or taken away*);
2. Make up for or make good (loss, damage, etc.);
3. Regain the strength, composure, balance, or the like, of oneself.

Recovery takes us back and to a previous place or state of where and what we once were. The problem with such an isolated meaning is that *we do not want to remain the same as we were* before we found cancer. If we "recover" to the same place, the same person with the same experiences, we will end up in the same current condition. Nothing changed to attack the root cause: it is still there!

To heal means:

1. To restore to *health* or soundness; *cure*;
2. To set right, repair;
3. To restore (a person) to spiritual wholeness.

There is much more to healing and health than the current Paradigm that modern Medicine addresses or offers. According to the New Cancer Paradigm, true healing cannot be achieved by treating only the body. We must also treat and heal the Mind. Millions of people have tried many different treatments and different therapies without getting the benefits they hoped.

Modern medical treatment is, of course, required, but it has created and propagated a mindset that mainly focuses only on the physical nature of the illness. It treats the symptoms or syndromes. When we have a headache, we take a pill. It might help the symptoms disappear for a while, but it does not heal the real source of the pain.

What causes the headaches? It could be allergies or it could be stress: it could be a pinched nerve, or a combination of many other things. The current Paradigm treats each *"thing" separately from every other "thing,"* but the New Cancer Paradigm collectively treats them all.

Immersive Healing

Immersive Healing is the new cancer Paradigm representing a revolutionary, breakthrough methodology for healing cancer and other chronic illnesses. Immersive Healing works alongside all current cancer treatments to improve recovery and outcomes for patients of all ages and with all types of cancer.

Medical treatment focuses only on the physical body. It treats the physical tumor independently of the rest of the body. Immersive Healing focuses on the *non-physical aspects of cancer* and heals the contributing factors that created the illness.

Throughout this book, I discuss and closely examine why focusing only on the body is simply not enough to bring about *true and real healing*. The Mind can affect the physical body by both creating illness and healing the illness.

Immersive Healing is a short, systematic method that can revive the innate healing mechanism already in place for healing. I share the scientific evidence for the development of this methodology and draw upon the work of both healers and scientists.

Heal the Source... Heal the Mind

To heal the Mind, the source of the deep-seated patterns of cancer must be found. Finding these patterns helps prevent cancer from resurfacing after the primary cancer is successfully treated by surgery, radiation, chemotherapy or other treatment. I offer a new perspective and a different way of healing your illness and interacting with it.

If you are with illness, healing the Mind provides the path to healing your body. A path and direction that mobilizes self-healing resources so your body can respond more effectively to your doctor's cancer treatment.

Immersive Healing focuses on the most overlooked location and aspect of the development of illness, *the powerful Subconscious Mind*. Healing the *non-physical aspects of* cancer means healing the deep-seated Mind Patterns that influenced the development of the illness in the first place. This allows the body's innate healing mechanisms to restore a state of health.

Researchers continue to explore and develop new treatments and therapies in an attempt to eliminate all cancers. Leading cancer research facilities worldwide continue to promote medical breakthroughs that revolutionize the treatment of cancer around the globe, but an end to the cancer epidemic is not in sight.

Immersive Healing Connects Modern Science to Modern Healing.

Immersive Healing is a short-term systematic therapeutic intervention designed to heal the root cause of the illness. It focuses on the mental patterns and Subconscious factors of the illness. Practiced as an adjunct to chemotherapy, surgery or radiation, Immersive Healing can and will help to: improve your quality of life, speed your recovery process and may reduce the amount of medication needed during treatment. It will also empower you to better cope with the side effects of your medical treatment. Immersive Healing makes you an active participant in your own healing process.

Immersive Healing is Safe and Drug Free

Immersive Healing is an advanced approach which is safe, drug free, painless, and non-invasive. It requires no hospital stay and no medication, and it has no side effects and no adverse effects on your quality of life. Immersive Healing is ultimately a freeing process.

Immersive Healing is used alongside conventional medical treatment to improve efficacy and outcome results.

Immersive Healing has Two Goals

"You can create a positive change in your body's ability to resist the cancer process." (Avinoam Lerner)

The primary goal of Immersive Healing is to heal the Mind Patterns believed to have initially produced the internal conditions for the cancer to develop. In the pages ahead, I discuss the Mind Model, and the relationship between the Conscious and Subconscious Mind. The secondary goal is to restore and strengthen the Immune System, the body's own natural defense system.

During the journey towards healing, it is reassuring to know that others have successfully traveled this road before you.

Many people believe cancer is caused by *a combination* of genetic, environmental, and psychological factors. Of far more importance than the cause *is what you can do about it*. We cannot alter the genetic factors, but we *can* alter the psychological influences by making "inner" changes that will transform your inner physical environment and change the conditions from which the cancer growth originated.

Nothing is Really Healed Until the Mind is Healed

Healing takes place when the Subconscious patterns suppressing the body's Immune System are resolved.

Prevention of illness can occur when the Subconscious Programming is healed. The Subconscious Mind is more powerful than you can ever imagine. *It can heal the illness as well as be the source of illness!*

Subconscious programming is not our fault! People around us, their words, comments, suggestion, unique circumstances and events that we had no control over, have programmed us from the time of our birth.

Events do not have meaning. Events only have meaning when we assign meaning to them. We assigned meaning to life events in an attempt to make sense of the world we live in so we can survive and function. Our responsibility and only measure of control is in our ability to *identify* (as adults) the faulty parts in our subconscious programming (i.e., distorted perceptions and self-limiting beliefs) that constitutes the Subconscious cry for self-mutilation or self-destruction and *choose* to *rewrite the program*. Although the focus of this book is cancer, illness is not the only way self-mutilation protocols manifest themselves. Addictions, harmful behaviors, and even destructive relationships are expressions of harmful programming.

If you are with cancer, it does not mean your Subconscious Programming is corrupt or bad. It is nothing like that, not at all! It does not mean your Subconscious Program is unusual or any worse than anyone else's.

We all grew up with different experiences in different habitats. Different *"things"* condition the Mind and we all have different manifestations of the programming. Each person's body is unique and each person's Subconscious is unique: that combination creates a unique experience.

The New Cancer Paradigm is *not* about having just a Mind-Body connection. The Mind-Body stuff out there still focuses on the *body*. I believe *you need to heal the Mind itself*. The New Paradigm takes us far beyond the Mind-Body connection. It is profoundly different from all the alternative healing methods out there for cancer. It goes much deeper than a simple Mind-Body connection.

Chapter 3

The Source and Origin of Health and Illness

Dr. Bruno Klopfer, the Psychologist who studied and reported Mr. Wright's remarkable recovery, was in fact studying to see if there was a *correlation between personality types and cancer growth rates*. Klopfer theorized that *certain personality types had faster or slower cancer growth rates than others*. He wanted to know if one personality experienced faster cancer growth while another type of personality would experience a slower growth rate.

His study was based on different personality types as they related to the type of cancer, age and other variables.

His initial theory was that p*eople with a high level of Ego drive would have less inner energy at their disposal to defend against the cancer,* and therefore the cancer would grow at a faster rate.

Mr. Wright had no chance to remain cancer free, according to Dr. Klopfer. Although his incredible Mind saved him twice, there was nothing to reinforce his belief. There was nothing in his personality that anchored further belief. In his words, "this could not last since it was not reinforced by any deep-rooted personality center with a long-range belief that could have counteracted the disastrous effect of his disappointment."

Dr. Klopfer knew something was missing from his theory and admitted the lack of practical application. So the question remained: What personality traits would have saved Mr. Wright? More importantly, how could he have acquired these personality traits?

Dr. Klopfer was primarily concerned with personality traits and their characteristics. I am intrigued by Kloper's theory of *thought patterns as a personality*. Our personality trait is a set of characteristics we outwardly reveal to the world. Klopfer concluded that there had to be something much deeper – a *"deep-rooted personality center"* beyond the reach of psychology that was a contributing factor to healing illness.

Our Multi-Dimensional Nature

Words used to describe a newborn child might be something like a five pound, blue-eyed girl, eighteen inches long with blond hair. At birth, we became a description of our physical body. As we grew older, we developed a personality, and inter-personal relationships. We became more than just the person we were at birth.

We learned how to think, developed reasoning skills, learned how to evaluate and experience emotions, to create and visualize, and to interact with others. While learning all of these things, we also developed a multi-dimensional reality of Mind and Body. We became a person from the combined experiences of three different dimensions: physical, psychological and spiritual.

Change and experience in one-dimension cause changes in another dimension. If we grew tall or were short (physical dimension) and felt as if we did not fit in, it may have affected the way we thought (Mind) and perceived ourselves. If we became overweight, we might have been teased and felt badly. An experience like this might have forced us to seek some form of spiritual guidance for comfort and self-survival. We may have also looked to other forms of inter-dimensional interaction to cope with the anxieties.

We felt *happy, euphoric, energized and excited* the first time we fell in love. These feelings translated physically into sweet anticipation and even a tingling sensation. We became deeply and spiritually connected because we discovered both the meaning and the purpose of being in love.

On the other hand, if we felt denied or rejected in some way, we became emotionally drained, lacked physical strength and felt spiritually withdrawn. Life seems to be without purpose or meaning when our inner world shrinks in this way. Think of the enormous amount of money spent every year treating anxiety and stress. According to CNN-Money.com, Americans spent more than $17 billion for anti-depressants and anti-anxiety drugs in 2010, up 10% from the previous year and nearly 30% over a two-year period. Now think of the impact all of this has on the physical body. Let there be no misunderstanding whatsoever about the impact and role the Mind plays in both our health and illness.

To explore our multi-dimensional constitution, I refer to the reasoning and logic of the late Viktor Frankl, M.D., Ph.D., a Professor of Neurology and Psychiatry at the University of Vienna (1905 – 1997)

Viktor Frankl's theory and therapy grew from his experiences as a prisoner in Nazi death camps. He concluded that philosopher Friedrich Nietzsche had it right: *"He who has a Why to live for can bear with almost any How."* (Nietzsche)

Frankl saw firsthand that people with hope, meaning and purpose survived more than those who had lost all hope, perceived the world meaningless, and had no purpose for living. People with hope of reuniting with loved ones and those with greater faith survived the challenges of the camp much better than those without.

Frankl's theory evolved into a form of *Existential Analysis* he called Logotherapy. As presented in his book *The Will to Meaning* (New American Library 1969),

Logotherapy offers a clear view of the possible spiritual dimension of cancer.

Logotherapy

One of the main assumptions of Frankl's Logtherapy is that human beings are spiritual (multi-dimensional) beings. Here the *implied* meaning of the word *"spiritual"* is stripped from any religious affiliation. Spiritual is used only within the scope of a secular concept representing the multi-dimensional nature of our being: physical (body), psychological (feelings and emotions) and spiritual (Mind).

We are aware mostly of our *physical dimension*. We know that we have a *psychological dimension*, but we often forget our spiritual dimension *that we can mobilize for healing*.

According to Frankl, problems arise when we project a multi-dimensional being onto a lower dimensional plane, such as the physical plane or psychological plane. When viewing a multi-dimensional person from only one-dimension, we miss valuable and vital information about the other dimension(s). In other words, we fail to see the whole or full composite of the person.

Frankl's Dimensional Ontology

Dimensional Ontology is a component of Logotherapy that logically explains the nature of perception. Frankl's laws of Dimensional Ontology provide an explanation of the way the human spirit relates to human science, especially the fields of psychology and Medicine.

It establishes the belief that humans are spiritual beings, thus multi-dimensional beings. By limiting the view of the human experience to a single dimension, we do not see the composite and complete Whole Person.

Frankl's First Law of Dimensional Ontology

"One and the same phenomenon projected out of its own dimension into different dimensions lower than its own is depicted in such a way that the individual pictures contradict one another (Figure 1)."

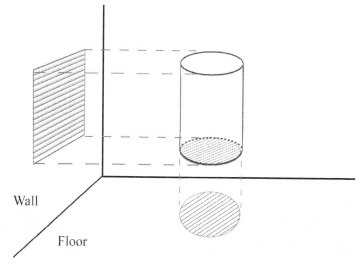

Wall

Floor

Figure 1

This is illustrated in Figure 1 which shows a cylinder suspended in a three-dimensional space. In the words of Frankl: "*Projected out of its three-dimensional space into the horizontal and vertical two-dimensional planes, it (the cylinder) yields in the first case a circle and in the second on a rectangle. These pictures contradict one another. What is more important, the cylinder is an open vessel* (open from the top, hollow) *in contrast to the circle and the rectangle that are closed figures."* (Will to Meaning)

In other words, the human experience has many dimensions: a *physical dimension* (rectangle), a *psychological dimension* (circle), and a *spiritual dimension* (the cylinder).

Each projection provides important information. The rectangle reveals its height and width, the circle reveals its circumference. However, neither one of these projections tells us that we are actually looking at a cylinder. We know it is a cylinder only because we can see the original object.

Neither projection informs us that the cylinder is, in fact, an open system, closed only at the bottom. Each projection provides limited information, and therefore we do not have a truly accurate or complete understanding of what the source object really is.

Why Frankl's Logic is Important to Cancer?

When it comes to understanding the human experience of illness, researchers have only studied cancer from a one-dimensional perspective. Based on Frankl's logic, researchers miss the real perspective, facts and important elements vital to treatment.

For example, medical practitioners view cancer as a physiological event taking place within the body. They only see cancer cells residing and dividing in the body, and their goal is to get rid of them!

By contrast, psychologists look at cancer through the lens of Mental Science in the context of social influences, behavioral patterns and certain personality types.

Each of these two projections provides important information, but each approach is extremely limited and incomplete. Each fails to see and thus treat the Whole

Person. Could this be the reason why we have not yet found the "cure" for the cancer? How can medical researchers find the cure if they only see cancer from the perspective of a singular dimension?

Despite almost inexhaustible resources, huge budgets, and unlimited manpower, no medical research study or doctor can definitively say what causes cancer with 100% scientific certainty. How could they with such a limited view of the problem?

Medical researchers discuss internal and external contributors. They can point to genetic disposition and carcinogenic factors in our environment. All true! But having cancer does not cause you to heal any better, so it is not good enough just to know that you have cancer and that it might be genetic. How does that create healing?

Viewing cancer treatment as a medical or biological event or only as a psychological event means robbing people of their true spiritual nature. It limits their experience to one or two dimensions, but we know that there are more dimensions.

Logotherapy assumes that humans are spiritual beings. This is very significant and missing from each of the other two dimensions. It is the spiritual dimension that provides meaning and purpose in one's life.

Continuing with Frankl's logic, we see that any attempt to completely cure cancer must include the spiritual dimension. The physical expression of cancer is the actual tumor. The tumor may respond well to chemotherapy, surgery, radiation treatment or psychotherapeutic intervention, but it *will not be "cured"* unless and until the *root cause* is also corrected and healed.

Origins of Illness: In Which Dimension Does Cancer Originate?

Now that we have established that human beings are multi-dimensional, the real question is obvious: In which dimension does cancer originate?

Frankl's Second Law of Dimensional Ontology

Frankl's second law provides evidence of the possibility that cancer can originate in the realm of the Subconscious Mind. It reads as follows: *"Different phenomena projected out of their own dimension into one-dimension lower than their own are depicted in such a manner that the pictures are ambiguous"* (Figure 2).

The three-dimensional objects -- *the cone, the cylinder and the ball* -- are all perceived as having the same shape when projected out of their three-dimensional world down on to a two-dimensional world (*the floor*), but in fact each object is distinctly different from each other.

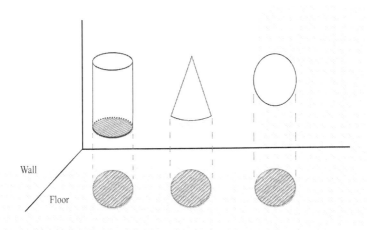

Figure 2

It is impossible to deduce the structure of the primary and true object simply by studying the shape each object casts on the floor. Figure 2 logically illustrates the importance of *perception* within the context of illness and cancer.

Let the circle on the floor represent a state of illness. Assume that each one of the original three-dimensional objects represents *a potential origin or source of illness*. Further we assume the physical and biological dimension of cancer is represented by the cylinder, the psychological dimension by the cone, and the realm of the Subconscious Mind (spiritual) by the ball.

There is only one logical conclusion. For some people, the cause of cancer is in the physical or biological dimension, for others the source lies within the psychological dimension, and for others it is in the realm of the Mind. How can you possibly begin to heal without treating all dimensions? You cannot! The answer is again as simple as the universal law of cause and effect, and it includes all dimensions!

The responsible thing to do is to recognize the possibility of illness originating in the realm of the Mind, the spiritual dimension.

By assuming that cancer is just a physical phenomenon or a psychological phenomenon, we fail to see the Whole Person. If we have only a limited view and cannot see the Whole Person, then we cannot treat the Whole Person. Therefore, we will fail to heal the Whole Person.

Obviously the physical, psychological, and spiritual dimensions must all be treated. Ignoring or waiting to take action on any dimension amounts to failing to take advantage of all the available options towards recovery. By failing to take action on all dimensions, we only partially treat the cancer. Why leave out a dimension in any cancer healing plan?

The result of such failure may lead to progression of cancer or its reoccurrence even in the face of the best Medicine has to offer. Why approach healing from such a limited perspective? You have everything to gain by treating all three dimensions.

Messages from Your Mind Echo in Your Body

Physical symptoms are tangible evidence of thought messages from your Subconscious Mind. Your body listens to your Mind and responds appropriately. These symptoms are representative of how we *really* feel deep inside. The body echoes what the Subconscious Mind (SM) tells it to do. Acne, skin rashes, etc., are common manifestations of intense emotional turmoil.

We pay very little attention to our body unless it is hurt or in pain. Then and only then do we pay full attention to what is taking place from within. When do you ever pay any attention to your back, legs, arms, shoulders or any other part of your body? *Only when it hurts!* You can see, touch, feel, experience and consciously observe a broken bone, a skin puncture, etc.

Do you ever think about your lungs, pancreas, kidneys, bladder or other part of your body? No, not consciously! Not unless you feel pain! A physical injury or accident is easy to diagnose and treat. The medical field is the appropriate method for treatment of most bodily injuries. Psychological wounds, trauma and destructive behavioral patterns can be identified as well. They are best treated within the realm of psychotherapy *and* the medical field.

A Wounded Mind

A Wounded Mind cannot be identified by looking at a chart, a scanner or picture. There is no x-ray to detect a Wounded Mind. We know something is wrong only when a significant change is taking place in our body. Typically, it is a change that we simply cannot ignore. Unlike an injured appendix, broken leg, hip replacement, etc., Mind Wounds cannot be treated with a surgical knife, medication or healed by the will power of the Conscious Mind.

Mind wounds are not in visible sight, but they are very much within us. Mind Wounds reside in the Subconscious Mind, between the tangible and intangible. These wounds represent a state of suppressed disharmony. Disharmony and discord are based on false meaning as a result of a limited personal view, erroneous perceptions and negative beliefs.

The Subconscious Mind is where we must look next if we are to leave no stone unturned on the journey towards improved health. This is the New Paradigm. A Mind Wound is the *intangible cause,* and cancer is its *tangible effect.* Healing the cause heals its effect.

Louise Hay in her book *Heal Your Body* offers insight into the mental pattern behind cancer. She describes the mental pattern of cancer as a *"deep hurt, longstanding resentment, deep secret of grief eating away at the self"*.

Take a moment to look within and review some of your most intimate thoughts. How do you honestly feel about yourself?

Become aware of your personal thoughts, those thoughts you think only in the privacy of your own Mind and ask yourself the following questions:

Are your thoughts filled with love, kindness and support? Are they all too often judgmental and critiquing? Do you practice cynicism and disdain? Do you offer yourself respect and reverence? Do you have a friend that can say the same things you say to yourself, and if so would you still be friends?

Cancer is often called the *disease of nice people*. That statement references the tendency of most people to hold their emotions inside rather than create a conflict.

In her book *Healing Happens with Your Help*, Carol Ritberger, Ph.D. wrote: "People who tend to have a higher predisposition to cancer seem to have patterns of behavior that encourage them to overextend themselves both mentally and emotionally for others, and who tend to put emotional needs of other people before their own."

Many of my clients identify with this statement. They often feel they have not lived authentically, having felt one way on the inside while acted differently on the outside. For example, you may agree to attend an event even though you know perfectly well that you are not one bit interested and would not enjoy it. You attend because you feel obligated.

This is not at all surprising, considering that we are taught not to say what we truly think and not to behave in a manner that reveals what we really think or feel. To do otherwise is viewed as inappropriate behavior.

These examples of harmonic dissonance create a state of disunity from within. They create the belief that we are not harmonically aligned and not in balance with our true authentic self.

If the Mind is Not in Harmony, Nothing Will Remain in Harmony!

Dissonance and discord are not our natural states of being. Life, nature and our world constantly strive for equilibrium.

The creative Subconscious Mind created the illness and used it as its vehicle and method to force us to make changes to restore a state of balance from within. It created pain and threat on a level that we could not deny, ignore, or afford to remain inactive. It forced our responsibility to take action.

You are called upon to take action in your life, to heal and live authentically. This will create an internal shift from imbalance to balance, from discord to harmony, and from illness to health.

Chapter 4

Heal the Mind, Heal the Cancer

The New Cancer Paradigm represents a fundamental shift in thinking about where, why and how the root cause and origin of cancer is healed. Illness is as serious as the Mind makes it out to be. Mind wounds have scars, not unlike the scars of physical wounds. Like physical scars, Mind Wounds must be healed in order for recovery and healing of the illness to take place. The New Cancer Paradigm draws its strength from our ability to control our mental activity and address and heal the disharmonious patterns promoting illness from within.

The way to treat and prevent cancer from returning is to eliminate its hidden root cause. For decades, medical researchers have worked relentlessly to find improved treatments and a cure to eradicate the cancer epidemic from only one-dimension.

Frankl's logic reminds us to think beyond the single *perception.*

Recall Mr. Wright's courage and conviction to try a new unknown treatment. He believed in the unfamiliar unknown treatment, and his belief renewed his physical health. He believed up until *the fear of failure* and negative news told him that the treatment would not work.

Armed with the wisdom of Viktor Frankl's Dimensional Ontology, we have a coherent and logical explanation about why we have not yet won the war on cancer. Frankl's logic is very simple: *researchers have been looking in the wrong place!* If we are to find a cure, it is imperative that researchers look beyond the two dimensions of biology or psychology. We must look into the realm of the Mind.

The words *brain and Mind* are often used interchangeably, but they are separate and different entities. The most noticeable difference is that the essence of the brain is physical, and the essence of Mind is spiritual. The brain is tangible, and the Mind is *in*tangible. The Mind is a field of consciousness involving thoughts, emotions, perceptions and beliefs. The brain is an organ inside the skull. It acts as a neural *"switchboard"* and the processor for our thoughts, emotions, perceptions and beliefs.

Think of your Mind as the architect and your brain as a builder. It is the builder's mission to convert the architect's plan into bricks and mortar.

New Beliefs, Biology, and DNA

Dr. Bruce Lipton is an internationally recognized authority whose studies bridge the scientific and the spiritual. A biologist by training, he taught cell biology at the University of Wisconsin School of Medicine, and then performed pioneering studies at Stanford University. His breakthrough research on the cell membrane in 1977 established the brand new science of epigenetics, the study of heritable changes in gene function that occur without a change in the DNA. His work provides remarkable evidence about how our thoughts and beliefs control the destiny of our living bodies.

At a cellular level, Dr. Lipton found that we possess innate intelligence which is far more crucial to shaping our lives than our genes. Prior to his research, biologists believed a "central dogma" that humans are biological bundles of chemical reactions at the sole direction of their own DNA. DNA scientists held the notion that we are a result of the DNA that we inherited and therefore are physically pre-programmed.

The new concept of epigenetics takes the position that it is our environment that controls our cells. Our thoughts and beliefs are an enormous part of our environment. The body consists of trillions of cells, and each one has a specific purpose, function, energy frequency, and digestive and elimination system.

Good health prevails when we have harmonic cells working together in a constant dialog, receiving the nutrients they need, kept safe from toxins, bacteria and viruses by the Immune System, and receiving healthy "signals" in the form of thoughts, emotions and beliefs. The old dogmatic approach left out the role of the environment.

Dr. Lipton found that cellular structure and function are very much inter-related. Every living organism has an information processor that interprets what goes on inside each cell. Our perception, thoughts and beliefs about our world and ourselves are signals that influence the cell data processor and affect the health of the cell. However, not all of our perceptions are accurate, and our biology is affected not only by our correct perceptions but also by our false perceptions.

The genes respond only to the perceptions of the cell, regardless of their validity. According to Dr. Lipton, our Conscious Mind processes about 40 bits of data per second, whereas our Subconscious Mind can process 40 *million* bits of data per second. Ninety percent of all our daily thoughts are sourced from our programmed Subconscious Mind.

Therefore, if we program thoughts such as *"I feel sick,"* that thought will become our reality and we will become sick. As much as seventy percent of the thoughts originating in our Subconscious Mind are repetitive and negative.

The Dichotomy of the Conscious & Subconscious Mind

The online encyclopedia states: "Common attributes of Mind include perception, reason, imagination, memory, emotion, attention, and a capacity for communication." The concept of a Dual Mind and its division to the Conscious and Subconscious Mind is perplexing.

We need to learn a little about the differences between the *Conscious Mind* and the *Subconscious Mind*. The dichotomy between our dual minds can produce a quandary: *consciously you want something and subconsciously you sabotage yourself from getting it.*

A Dual Mind System refers to our unique ability to be *"of two minds"* and is the gateway to the root cause of illness. The Subconscious Mind and the Conscious Mind can run different programs at the same time, one negative and one positive.

Successful singers, actors and other celebrities are examples of this reality. They stood in the limelight and it became too bright. Celebrities were admired by so many and believed to have certain qualities and attributes like confidence and competency. They dressed provocatively, appeared happy, and gave the world the impression they possessed all the positive things life had to offer. Unfortunately we later read in their memoires about their struggles and personal daemons such as insecurity and poor self-image.

During casual conversations, we use the word *Mind* to refer to both the Conscious and Subconscious. The dichotomy of a Dual Mind explains how illness can subconsciously develop below the surface of our consciousness, while at the same time we can feel consciously intact, positive and healthy.

The Conscious and Subconscious Minds

At the risk of oversimplifying such a sophisticated mechanism as the Mind, I use the *Human Mind Model*. It helps to explore the terrain of the Mind in a similar way that a road map helps us find our way in an unfamiliar city or country.

Gerald F. Kein, a noted hypnotist from the Omni Hypnosis Center in Florida, developed the Human Mind Model (Figure 3). It is a useful way to clarify the functional purposes of the Conscious Mind and Subconscious Mind. It also explains how Subconscious Programming occurs.

The Mind consists of three agencies: the *Conscious Mind, Subconscious Mind and Unconscious Mind.* My focus is mainly on the *interaction between the Conscious Mind and Subconscious Mind* and the ability of each to *influence* health and healing. The Unconscious Mind is excluded from this particular Mind Model discussion due to the nature of its *autonomic* mental phenomena. The autonomic functions include instincts and autonomic bodily functions (breathing, heartbeat, body temperature, etc.) These processes are beyond the scope of our therapeutic intervention, and therefore add little value to our understanding of the Mind.

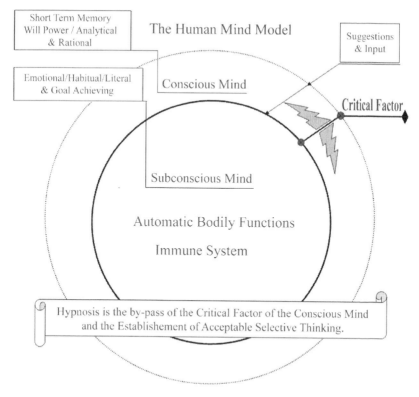

Figure 3

The Conscious Mind – The Rational Mind

The outer ring of the Mind Model in Figure 3 represents the Conscious Mind, also referred to as the *rational Mind* or the *critical Mind*. Will power and short-term-memory reside in the Conscious Mind. I characterize the Conscious Mind as rational and analytical, with the ability to:

- Look, Listen and Learn
- Reason and Judge

- Analyze and Criticize
- Accept and/or reject

Two of the main *"jobs"* of the Conscious Mind are to:

1. *Alert us of any potential threat* to our physical or emotional safety.

2. *Guard against inconsistencies* of our current thought Paradigm. It serves to filter external input, such as words, ideas, suggestions and data processed via our five senses.

Using this oversimplified analogy, we can think of the Subconscious Mind as a *"memory" bank* and the Conscious Mind as the *"bank" guard*. Like a guard that protects the gold in the vault at Fort Knox, the Conscious Mind guards and protects the information stored in the Subconscious Mind. In this case, the guard's job has nothing to do with the actual *"gold"* inside the vault (memories, beliefs, perceptions, etc.). Its only function is to allow those with the proper security clearance to have access or get in.

The Subconscious Mind – The Emotional Mind

The inner ring of the Mind Model illustration represents the Subconscious Mind. Unlike the *rational and critical* Conscious Mind, the Subconscious Mind is characterized as *emotional and habitual*.

The Subconscious Mind's primary role is to seek and actively attain *homeostasis*, a balanced emotional, mental, and physical state, a role in which we have little conscious participation. Ever watchful, it *monitors and interprets* our *mental, emotional, or physical* state. It communicates our deeper needs in the form of *feelings and sensation* that provide information about our internal environment.

The Subconscious Mind performs the following functions:

1. Run all bodily systems necessary for sustained physical life (those not controlled consciously), such as digestion, the beating of the heart, breathing, etc.

2. Harbor perceptions, beliefs, ideas, concepts and information received via the five senses.

3. Act out and create or make real in our lives conditions based on our perception, beliefs, ideas and concepts.

Envision your Subconscious Mind as a library, a private library of books filled with only information about your life. Think of the books as a series entitled *This is Your Life*. Each book represents a period in your life, and each page in each book is an interpretive encyclopedia of your life events and experiences. Every moment in our lives is perceived via input from our five senses: touch, taste, smell, sound and hearing. The perceived impressions from our senses are "recorded" and stored in this library. Our senses receive external input and convert them into memory data banks. The information now in memory is available and ready for recall and review.

Stephen Parkhill describes the Subconscious Mind as *"The most powerful goal achieving agency known to men."* I have augmented that description of *the Subconscious Mind* to include its ability to turn the *invisible to visible, thoughts to actions, ideas and concepts into things,* and *beliefs into conditions*. We create our own reality by embracing specific attitudes and beliefs we have come to know as our own. The Subconscious Mind relentlessly strives to produce physical expressions and conditions based on those beliefs and perceptions.

This means we must *"be"* before we can *"do"*, and we can *"do"* only to the extent that we *"are,"* and what we *"are"* depends upon what we *"think."* (Charles F. Hannel)

The *goal-seeking faculty of the Subconscious Mind* will not function until there is an *"established point"* of relativity. The very *first messages* ever received into the Subconscious Mind, about any subject, topic, or idea, were placed into permanent memory. These first messages became the *"established point"* of relativity to all future messages. It makes no difference if the first perception was correct or incorrect, good or bad. The first impression in the Subconscious Mind was formed simply because *it was the first message ever placed in the Subconscious Mind's memory.* That first message became the perception from which *all other messages* were considered for acceptance or rejection into the Subconscious Mind.

The first message *was free from any filtering by the Conscious Mind, free from any judgment, and uncensored.* It was placed in permanent memory. The Mind had now established *a starting point* and a perception about that subject or topic. All new and future messages were relative to the "established first" perception. Evidence of the ability of the Subconscious Mind to manifest itself is pervasive and overwhelming.

If we accept the fact that every man-made product was first drawn on the canvas of the Subconscious Mind and each one began as a thought or idea before it could be manufactured, then we must also accept that every other aspect of our life was first a mental impression, including the state of our health and well-being, a belief or perception in the Subconscious Mind.

The Literal Nature of the Subconscious Mind

The Subconscious Mind is powerful and omnipotent, but is unable to bear *judgment* on the information it harbors. It is completely literal, *rendering no opinion or judgment as to the quality or type of information, negative or positive beliefs, false or real perceptions.*

The Subconscious Mind believes exactly what it is told. All programmed beliefs, whether harmful, negative, and false, or healthy and positive, become the literal truth. The Subconscious Mind does not have the ability to judge or reason about anything; it cannot determine what messages are good or bad.

The Subconscious Mind is vulnerable and needs protection. The Conscious Mind provides the necessary protection by filtering and critiquing the information entering the Subconscious Mind.

Imagine what would happen if the Conscious Mind's protection mechanism did not exist! If I told you that 2 + 2 = 7, the Subconscious would accept this as literal truth. A moment later I might suggest that 2+2 = 48, and the Subconscious would once again accept my literal words as truth. Without the capacity to reason, judge, compare or establish relationships to what you already know, the literal nature of Subconscious Mind would be in constant chaos.

Taste the Lemon

Here is a simple exercise that will show firsthand the literal nature of your Subconscious Mind. This simple and short exercise uses your Mind's imagination to demonstrate the power of the Mind-Body relationship. It establishes the foundation of logic as to how the physical body can respond to thoughts, and how thoughts can be used to heal your illness.

Begin the exercise by imagining you are holding a fresh, ripe, yellow juicy lemon in your hand. Visualize the lemon in every possible way, and in your mind's eye give the lemon a little squeeze just to confirm how very ripe and juicy it is. Hold that clear and vivid mental picture in your Mind. If imagination and visualization do not work for you, then think instead of the smell of the lemon and its sour taste. Concentrate on the brilliant bright yellow color, the shape, texture, smell, lemonade, lemon scents, squirting juice, and the smell of its skin.

When you have the mental picture and thoughts of a lemon, pretend you hold a lemon in one hand, and then imagine slowly cutting the lemon in half. Because it is so very juicy, the juice squirts everywhere as you cut it.

Now imagine holding half the lemon in your hand... visualize it as vividly as you can... feel the rough texture and imagine the juice sparkling on the flesh of the lemon... oh so ripe... you can smell the scent of the lemon as you bring the juicy, sour lemon to your mouth and lips.

Now open your mouth wide and squeeze all the sour juice into your mouth, swish it around for a moment while savoring its taste, and notice its effect!

What is happening inside your mouth? Did you feel the tingling sensation in your mouth? Did you salivate? When done right, you will have these feelings and sensations.

The simple lemon exercise quickly and effectively demonstrates the Mind-Body phenomenon at work. Your body responds to thoughts, mental images, and visualization you create and hold in your Mind. An existing perception (of a lemon) programmed into the Subconscious Mind *can and will* produce the proper physical response (salivation) and condition.

The existing perception of what a lemon looks like and what it tastes like was then converted into mental images that in turn signaled a physical response within the body. It processed a lemon as it understood the perception of a lemon to be.

The Literal Discipline of the Subconscious Mind

The lemon exercise demonstrates the very important literal discipline of the Subconscious. Think about what this exercise proved! Without a real lemon in your hand and without tasting even one drop of real lemon juice, your physical mechanism kicked in and responded just as if you had a real lemon in your hand! This is an amazing and very powerful exercise.

Your Subconscious Mind did not care that the entire event took place *only* in your imagination. To the Subconscious Mind it was very real, and that's also why your body responded as if it were a real event. Your mind and body thought the lemon event was real.

This exercise provides a personal firsthand experience of the relationship between your Mind and Body. The Mind-Body relation is now a firsthand experience, no longer just a theory but a proven fact. You just experienced one of the most important aspects of the Mind-Body relationship, how a thought can create a physical response and experience.

The same mechanism that converted your thoughts into a physical response is the mechanism involved in forming illness or bringing about your health!

The Iceberg Metaphor

Another good analogy of the relationship between the Conscious and Subconscious is the iceberg metaphor. The originator of this analogy was none other than Dr. Sigmund Freud (1856-1939) considered the father of psychotherapy and the creator of psychoanalysis.

That portion of the iceberg above the water's surface (Figure 4) is analogous to the Conscious Mind which by some accounts represents about 10% of our thinking ability. The Subconscious Mind accounts for the other 90% represented by the large mass below the water's surface.

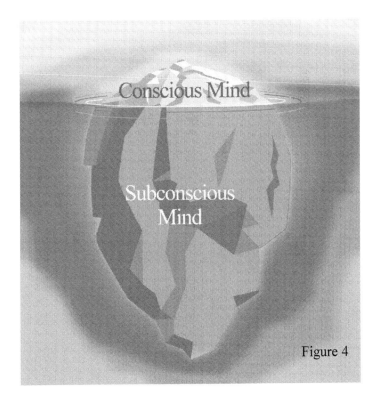

Figure 4

Harmony and Disharmony in the Mind

We have learned to observe *good health as a state of harmony and balance* within, and *illness as a state of out of balance or disharmony.*

Subconscious Paradigms function as the body's blueprints for either health or illness. Subconscious Paradigms are energetic designs or bodies of mental information that influence physiology and bodily functions. Every thought and emotion has its own energetic signature or vibration frequency.

The frequency of the energy wave is altered when we change the way we think and feel. Essentially, we have the ability to transform our thoughts and feelings in a way that will invalidate and cancel a previous pattern and its effect. For example, think of the word *stress*. Now take a moment and think about the word *relaxation*. Allow yourself to feel the contradicting effect within, and how one sensation tends to cancel the other.

Do the same with the words *panic and calm, shame and pride.* Each of these *"word thoughts"* carry information that influences the way you feel and behave. We all create our world through observations and the resulting perceptions. These perceptions become our truths to the extent that we assign meaning to events.

How do we rewrite programs in our Subconscious Mind?

Immersive Healing provides a method to override our existing Subconscious programs. This approach recognizes the Dual Mind system and heals the rift between the two minds.

As Lipton explained, DNA is not solely responsible for steering our biological ship. DNA is influenced by *"information" originating in the Mind in the form of beliefs, thoughts and emotions.* Thoughts and emotions by themselves cannot cause or cure cancer, but they do affect our body chemistry. Biochemistry affects the development and environment for cancer to develop. As our body chemistry affects feelings, it also creates a physical response.

Beliefs are ideas, concepts, rules and assumptions incorporated into our lives which we hold to be true. They are true to us because of repeated situations that seem to "prove" their legitimacy. Beliefs shape our thoughts, attitudes and behavior.

The brain communicates "information" to the rest of the body using an extensive network of neurons. Neurons send messages electrochemically that cause an electrical signal, an energy surge. Everything in the universe has energy and vibrates at a certain frequency. As humans we constantly create and receive waves of energy. Conventional Medicine uses this knowledge every day. For example, a lung x-ray is a picture of the vibration energy diagrams of lung cells.

Our thoughts form the information in our energy vibration. A thought becomes a belief when you have convinced yourself that it is valid. Once programmed into the Subconscious Mind, it affects a big part of your life.

Illness is a reflection of a state of disharmony *within*. Fear is the first instinctive reaction, but fear does not create healing. Fear can lead to avoidance and denial: it serves only to strengthen the current state of illness.

Think of the body as the delta of a river. The flowing water represents your Mind's energy. When the water is full of nutrients, farmers can grow healthy crops. Residents in the towns along the river get fresh, clean drinking water to maintain and support their state of health. However, if the quality of the water becomes poor or contaminated, the crops die and the town's people will be forced to search for a new supplemental source of drinking water.

The river analogy helps to understand the above statement about how the quality of the Mind's energy will affect our body as it flows throughout. Thoughts, emotions and beliefs are forms of energy that flow through the body via the central nervous system.

We must find the source of "contamination" in the flow of energy in order to regain health and heal.

Chapter 5

The Subconscious Illness Paradigm

With insight into the function and purpose of the Subconscious Mind, we can begin to study the role it plays in illness. Specifically, we learn how Subconscious Paradigms are created and how an Illness Paradigm contributes to the development of cancer.

Previously I referenced the *non-physical aspects of illness,* i.e., the integral Subconscious components that form the Subconscious Illness Paradigm (SIP).

The online dictionary defines Paradigm as *"A set of assumptions, concepts, values, and practices that constitute a way to view reality for the community that shares them."* This definition is very much in line with what is called the Conditioning Process as outlined in Figure 5.

A Subconscious Paradigm is *the sum of our perceptions, concepts and beliefs we have formed about the world and ourselves throughout our lives.* Contrary to our beliefs, our actions and reactions are not the result of logical and systematic thought processes. They are byproducts of our Conditioning Process and can be traced back to birth when the Subconscious Mind was first forming.

The term "Conditioning Process" refers to an ongoing learning process. Learning may occur consciously or without conscious awareness through interaction with others, play, repetition and association. It is by this process that we come to "know" *our world.*

A classic way to teach (condition) young children about animals is to match and pair an animal with its sound, i.e., *"what sound does a cow make?"* Most authorities agree that the conditioning process is largely completed by the age of six. As Brian Tracy defines it: *"our self-concept"* is set, meaning our perception of self is already defined.

During our formative younger years, we are always functioning in a *"receiving"* Mind mode. Everything we perceived from our five senses and learned from those around us helped shape an understanding of who we are. It also shapes how the world operates with us in it (more or less).

I am speaking of all experiences, everything we have ever heard, ever seen, smelled, touched, tasted and learned, intentionally or unintentionally, as *suggestions.*

Reality is a subjective experience based on our interpretation of an experience, rather than the ultimate or absolute truth of the experience. It is our interpretation of the experiences and *not* the absolute truth of those experiences that become our reality.

Within the context of illness and health, it is important to understand that *all input processed from our five senses is considered as suggestions*. While sight and hearing are obvious, touch, taste and smell also have a profound impact on our perceptions.

The Conditioning Process, Success & Failure

We need to understand the Conditioning Process and how Subconscious Programming takes place. We can begin to see how comments and *suggestions* (some innocent and some not) build into a thought Paradigm that affects our lives.

A child is more likely *to believe* someone he or she depend on for all aspects of their well-being, someone who feeds, clothes and loves them. We do not arrive on this earth with a user's manual to show us how to survive and exist. When it comes to learning new skills, we depend on others.

Whether we are aware of it or not, we are constantly learning. Suggestions we hear, repeated and compounded over a period of years, grow into our belief system. Our beliefs shape our attitudes and outlook. *Negative beliefs form negative attitudes, and positive beliefs form positive attitudes.*

Our attitude is like a color prism of our lives. A negative attitude paints our world in dull colors and shades. Negative attitudes become self-fulfilling prophecies because they become our truth. With a negative attitude and view of ourselves, we avoid opportunities, do not stand up for ourselves, and do not pursue our dreams. We become critical, judgmental and have difficulty making changes. Focusing on the negative results in despair, hopelessness and failure.

Attitudes influence thoughts, and thoughts are reflected in our behavior. Successful thoughts lead to success, and thoughts of failing lead to more failure. Eventually, our dominant thoughts will become our *Thought Paradigm.*

The Thought Paradigm creates a *Mind fence* with an invisible barrier of fear. Fear inhibits personal growth! Lack of personal growth cements our limited self-view into our identity. This explains why so many people go through life only to experience the same set of circumstances, conditions and results they already know.

We tend to recreate what is already familiar even if it is negative. We do so because *it is familiar and makes us feel more secure.* In the hierarchy of human needs and values, safety and security are at the top of the list.

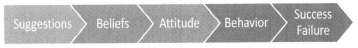

External expression of the Conditioning Process: Figure 5

Case Study: Joe - Prostate Cancer

This case study of one of my clients highlights the power of the Conditioning Process. I will call this client Joe. As a child, Joe grew up in a home hearing negative suggestions on a daily basis. He constantly heard suggestions like: *"You make me so mad," "you are useless," "I am so disappointed in you," "I can't believe you did this to me," "why can't you be more like your brother," "stop being such a baby for God's sake, be a man,"* and many other negative statements.

Those suggestions were repeated so often that Joe accepted and believed them to be true. After all, they were made by the ultimate authority figures in his life, *his parents*. Joe believed his parents were not pleased with anything about him. These negative messages made him feel inadequate in their eyes. Whatever he did was wrong, not good enough, disappointed his parents, or had consequences and punishment.

Joe was a child and therefore did not have the "reasoning" ability of an adult. He began to accept all of these negative statements as fact.

His beliefs blossomed into a negative and self-defeating attitude. That attitude was reflected in everything he tried to do. Joe's thought process *was trapped* in a vicious cycle of thoughts and their expressions. Each failure brought him closer to the view that: *"I can't, I won't, I am not,"* etc. Over a period of time the words that gave birth to his negative beliefs became his own words and added fuel to his self-defeating attitude and negative self-thoughts.

As a child Joe had no *logical reasoning ability or inner-voice to counter attack* the *"evidence"* at hand. His negative view of himself led to the failure of his business as an adult and later blossomed into his illness.

If Joe had received positive suggestions and positive reinforcement suggestions such as: *"you can do anything you set your Mind to," "you are so smart," "I'm so proud of you," "I know you can do it," "keep trying Joe, you are learning,"* etc., his thought Paradigm would inevitably have been positive and would have led to success.

A *positive self-view*, reinforced with positive words from Joe's parents such as *"I can, I shall, I will"* would have brought about very different results.

Following the programming instructions outlined in Figure 6, it is likely that Joe would have felt more confident, with more self-worth and more determination to pursue and overcome challenges both personally and with his business. Such a pursuit for happiness and success is the birthright for every one of us.

The Conditioning Process, Illness & Health

Now that we understand how the Conditioning Process or "Subconscious Programming" affects behavior, success and failure, let's further investigate its effect on our health. As I previously discussed, *our beliefs create our reality.* However, this time *the belief* is in the form of an Illness Paradigm. Subconscious Illness Paradigm is composed *thought by thought*, day by day, week by week and so on.

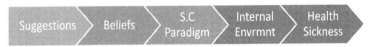

Internal Expression of the Conditioning Process: Figure 6

If the Subconscious Mind harbors beliefs about self-worth, beliefs from which it forms an attitude that translates to success or failure, it can hold beliefs about whether or not we are *worthy of health* or *worthy of sickness.*

An active Subconscious Illness Paradigm brings about a level of stress that causes a chain reaction within the physical body. A high level of stress causes the brain to produce and inject stress hormones into the blood stream such as Adrenaline and Cortisol.

The long-term activation of the stress-response system and subsequent overexposure to stress hormones *disrupt almost all of our body's processes.*

Harmful Beliefs & Perceptions	Accumulated Stress	Chemical Toxicity	Physical & Emotional Symptoms	Chronic Conditions, Cancer

The Conditioning Process, Stress & Illness: Figure 7

Change at the level of belief and perception will lead to change in their expression. Harmful beliefs flourish as illness, positive beliefs flourish as health.

Our priority is to identify those harmful beliefs and perceptions that form the Subconscious Illness Paradigm, and then replace them with beliefs and perceptions that will promote health from within.

Joe interpreted all the negative suggestions he heard so many times as "it's all my fault," "I am responsible for my parents' unhappiness," and "if I were not here they would have been better off." He viewed himself as a source of irritation for his parents and the cause of their pain and unhappiness.

As children we had limited use of our mental and emotional faculties because they were still in the process of developing. Children are unable to "rationalize" situations as adults, understand the big picture, or evaluate things that are said as to whether they are true, false, or right or wrong. Children tend to accept everything they are told as being true.

We paint our world in absolute colors rather than shades. This serves to reinforce ideas and beliefs we already have established about ourselves and, in the case of illness, deepen the Mind Patterns that created it in the first place.

The Mind: Health and the Law of Vibration

"Everything is a vibration and its effect. In actuality, no physical matter can exist. All the physical matters are composed of vibration." (Dr. Max Planck, Nobel Prize in Physics).

The Subconscious Mind communicates information in the form of feelings and emotions. Each feeling, thought and emotion has its own unique vibration and wavelength, similar to how each musical instrument vibrates to create sounds. Emotions such as fear, grief and despair vibrate at a low frequency, while feelings such as love, joy and gratitude vibrate at a higher frequency.

Everything in nature has a rate of vibration, including the human body. The body is a mass of molecules vibrating at a very high frequency. Not only is the body receptive, it is physically affected by the frequency of vibration.

Data from the Subconscious Mind (SCM) communicates directly with the brain. The brain receives and processes the data, then sends it on to the rest of the body via the central nervous system. Data travels in the form of a vibration. Each data transmission modifies and alters the vibration in every atom, cell, and organ in the body.

The Law of Vibration states that: "Everything in the universe is what it is by virtue of its rate of vibration. Change the rate of vibration and you change the nature, quality, and form. The vast panorama of nature, both visible and invisible, is being constantly changed by simply changing the rate of vibration, and as thought is a vibration, we can exercise this power. We can change the vibration and thus produce any condition that we desire to manifest in our bodies." (Charles F. Hannel).

The Sound of the "Wounded" Mind

Imagine your brain as an orchestra, and your beliefs, perceptions, emotions and attitudes as musical instruments. Each instrument vibrates at a specific frequency to create a unique sound.

If you could listen to the soundtrack of your Subconscious Mind, what would it sound like? Would you hear harmonious or disharmonious sounds in your orchestra?

When illness is present, the sound is not harmonious. In this case, the vibration generated by the orchestra in our Subconscious Mind is one of disharmony.

Harmful beliefs, erroneous perceptions and unresolved emotional turmoil fuel the Subconscious Illness Paradigm to generate disharmonious vibrations, and we become ill. In a state of illness, the soundtrack of your subconscious mind would be like an orchestra of untrained musicians playing un-tuned instruments.

Without being aware of what we are doing, we "think" ourselves into illness because our thoughts, beliefs and emotions affect the body. The model in Figure 8 illustrates how Mind factors affect our brain and our body.

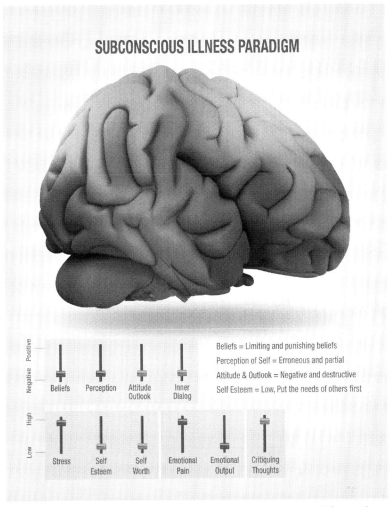

Figure 8

Harmonizing the Subconscious Mind

We can "think" ourselves back into good health. We have the ability to change the Subconscious Paradigm from *one of illness* to *one of health*. To get the Subconscious Mind back into a harmonic state of health, we must identify, address and heal every aspect of the Subconscious Illness Paradigm that is not in harmony. We must change the beliefs and perceptions from negative to positive.

"The way to health is founded on the law of vibration, which is the basis of all science, and this law is brought into operation by the Mind, the 'world within'. It is a matter of individual effort and practice. Our world of power is within. If we are wise, we shall not waste time and effort in trying to deal with effects as we find them in the 'world without', which is only an external, a reflection." (Charles F. Hannel)

Immersive Healing is a method for changing Disharmonious Mind Patterns (DMP) to Harmonious Mind Patterns (HMP). The DMP created illness in the first place. By changing from DMP to HMP, we change from destructive to constructive, become courageous and allow healing to begin. Discord, disharmony, and disease give way to mental, psychological and physical health (Figure 9).

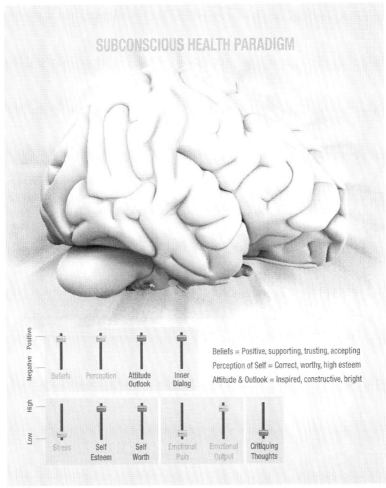

Figure 9

Immersive Healing is not the only path to restoring harmonious Mind Patterns. Self-help gurus promote the use of affirmations. Affirmations are declarations of desired ideas and outcomes. Such declarations repeated over and over again saturate the *Conscious Mind* and impress the *Subconscious Mind* with a new directive. Over a period of time, the new directive can influence and change our beliefs. This process requires a lot of time, effort, concentration and persistence. Unfortunately many cancer patients do not have the time it takes.

The affirmation process may also be opposed by the Critical Faculty of the Conscious Mind which strongly protects your Subconscious Illness Paradigm. Focus, confidence and tenacity is required to penetrate the Critical Faculty. In the case of chronic illness and cancer, this requires a systematic therapeutic process such as Immersive Healing which uses hypnosis as the main therapeutic vehicle.

Hypnotherapy is the practice of using hypnosis for the purpose of therapeutic intervention. While Hypnotherapy is *not the only way* to make changes on the Subconscious level, it provides a clear path to the Subconscious Mind while bypassing the Critiquing Faculty of the Conscious Mind.

The Initial Sensitizing Event (ISE)

The Initial Sensitizing Event (ISE) is a specific moment when an external *event* profoundly *altered* our self-perception in a negative way. It is the *seed of illness* planted in the fertile ground of our Subconscious Mind. The *alteration in perception* is "seen" by the Subconscious Mind as the seed planting or the *origin* of a problem, symptom or condition.

Spiritual doctrines have long referenced defining moments and events that changed mankind. The biblical description of the expulsion from the Garden of Eden is a well-known example. Other doctrines define such a moment as the as the moment of separation from God, the Universe or Oneness.

I see illness as *the blooming seed of the moment of separation planted in the vulnerable mindset during the early formative years.* The ISE holds the key to all healing and, therefore, the key to health. Healing the "moment of separation" requires restoring awareness and repairing our perception of self. Immersive Healing can change a negative and fractured perception to one of *positive and wholeness.*

In Search of Your ISE

We are the authors of our own individual life experiences. Even though *we are not responsible* for all the experiences that happened during our childhood, *we perceived and interpreted* all of those events. Therefore, we became the author of our life experiences,

A wise friend once told me that: *"events in and of themselves have no meaning, they have consequences."* We assign meaning to our events for the purpose of survival as we attempt to make sense of our world.

An objective observer may see an event in our lives as a sequence of actions. We may have interpreted and labeled those actions as negative or positive, pleasant or unpleasant, helpful or harmful. However, these are *our own interpretations and no one else's.* Just as fingerprints are distinct to each individual, interpretations of life's events are distinctly ours.

Events elicit emotions and feelings. Events we interpret as positive elicit positive emotions and feelings, whereas those events we interpret as negative elicit negative emotions and feelings.

In the context of cancer, we must focus on those erroneous perceptions and the negative feelings and emotions they produced that formulated the

Subconscious Illness Paradigm. Healing the root cause of the Subconscious Illness Paradigm, the ISE, also heals all of its expressions, *illness included.*

In his book *Answer Cancer – The Healing of a Nation*, Steve Parkhill discusses the importance of the ISE in healing by using the illustration showing an inverted pyramid of cans in Figure 10. His model is invaluable in its simplicity and accuracy.

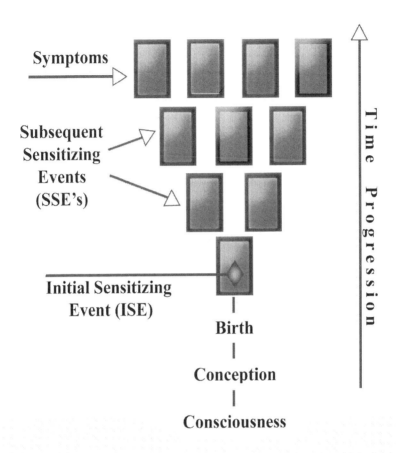

Figure 10

The cans in the top row graphically represent symptoms of known illnesses. Proper treatments are selected to mute the symptoms by altering the body's chemistry and biology. Chemotherapy, surgery and radiation are the weapons of choice for treating cancer.

The next two rows represent the compounding life events, the Subsequent Sensitizing Events (SSE's) that coagulate and cement the Illness Paradigm. The nature of these events is psychological and, therefore, the usual treatments include psychotherapy and/or psychiatry.

The single can at the bottom represents the ISE, *that moment in time when our perception of our world and of ourselves changed.* At that moment, our perception changed from pure, good and whole (*the attributes of consciousness*) to tainted, negative and fractured (*the attributes of Ego*). This is when we first learned that negativity has meaning.

Prior to the ISE, there is birth. Prior to birth, there is the moment of conception. What came before the moment of conception is what we must consider within the scope of the Healing Paradigm. While each school of thought refers to them by different names, i.e., God, love, universe, etc., the one thing they all have in common is that they all tend to agree to its *nature* as *pure, good and whole.*

In terms of Viktor Frankl's second law of Dimensional Ontology discussed in Chapter 3, the top row of cans in Figure 10 represents the physical dimension, the next two rows represent the psychological dimension, and the single can at the bottom represents the realm of the Subconscious Mind.

Many of my clients have previously participated in one or more forms of psychotherapy. Some gained insight into the terrain of their emotional landscape, and others learned valuable and beneficial coping skills. Despite these benefits, the majority of my clients say they feel unchanged from within.

To Every Effect There is a Cause

We know *that to every effect there is a cause.* However *not every ISE becomes active.* In other words, planting seeds in the ground does not ensure that a tree will grow for each seed. In order for the seed to germinate and grow, it needs water and nourishment.

An ISE can only germinate into a full blown Subconscious Illness Paradigm when its underlying message is compounded repeatedly. Like the perception of illness, nourishment for an ISE comes in the form of repetition and reinforcement of the harmful perception born in it. These reinforcing events are called Subsequent Sensitizing Events or SSE.

It may surprise you to realize the ISE need not be an event equivalent to the *Big Bang*, dramatic or of epic proportion. Most often the ISE is not even consciously remembered.

Rather than a traumatic event, the ISE can be an ordinary every day event, a casual exchange of words, a comment or a conclusion that impressed your Mind with negativity.

Subsequent Sensitizing Events (SSE)

As the name suggests, a Subsequent Sensitizing Event (SSE) is *any event that reinforces and compounds an existing perception.* In the context of illness and the Subconscious Illness Paradigm, SSE reinforced a negative underlying message buried in the ISE.

For example, a child falls repeatedly when learning to ride a bicycle. Falling this way is expected and, therefore, causes no lasting emotional impact. However, one day the neighborhood kids see the child fall and they all laugh, point and tease. The child responds emotionally with shame, rejection and fear. This event becomes the ISE. The ISE stated inadequacy, social ridicule and rejection.

Two years later, the same child mispronounces words while reading a short story in front of classmates. Once again, the child is ridiculed and teased by the other children. This event triggered an already existing emotional pattern of shame, and fear stored in the ISE.

If the ISE is the *seed planting* of negative self-view and harmful beliefs, the SSE provide the nourishment for the seed to fully bloom as an illness. Just like the seeds of tree need nourishment, the SSE has now become the nourishment for ISE.

SSEs are emotional by nature, not intellectual. Their emotional nature makes a strong enough impact for the door to the Subconscious Mind to open wide.

The Power of Words to Hurt or Heal

Words are powerful. They can inspire peace between nations or summon warriors to war. Words can inspire love, peace, hate, war, motivation, harmony, and health, or they can call for punishment and scorn. *Words have the power to heal the body or harm the body!*

Words spoken by someone else or spoken from our "inner dialog" have the power to heal or the power to make us ill. We create the truth because we assign meaning to our experience, just as Mr. Wright did when he assigned truth to the drug he believed would cure him. We create the world through our observations and the resulting perceptions.

Negativity, criticism and ridicule have immense power over our experience, as do words of praise, support, confidence and love.

A child who hears a negative statement *once* is not likely to experience harmful negative long-term beliefs. However, repeated frequent negative statements will hurt a child, especially if spoken by a figure of authority at a critical moment. This is especially true if those words were delivered with cynicism and ridicule at that critical moment of vulnerability.

A critical moment is any moment of "Mind Innocence" when a child has no judgment and cannot evaluate or rationalize the meaning of the spoken words. The child's ears absorb the spoken word as if they are the only active part of the body during that moment. Having not yet learned to analyze the meaning of the words, the child believes them. The ears heard those words and, therefore, the child believes the words.

During early formative years, we are completely dependent on adults. We have blind trust and absolute belief in everything adults say, having not yet learned to exercise rational or critical thinking. Adults and children have a hypnotic contract without being consciously aware of its presence. The door to the Subconscious Mind opens wide and words affect change.

Positive words build self-esteem, generate energy and vitality, and in so doing promote health. Negative and toxic words build limiting negative beliefs, deplete our physical energy, and create the conditions for illness to develop within our body.

The Birth of Incorrect Perception

In the context of the Subconscious Mind (SCM), the expression *"you only get one chance to make a first impression"* is the ultimate truth. Perception in the Subconscious Mind follows the rule of *first come first served.* The first perception to enter the SCM is automatically *accepted without judgment.* The first perception will stay there until removed. That perception becomes the model of reality from which every other experience is measured.

This holds true whether or not the perception is correct, incorrect, positive, or negative. Once accepted, that perception remains in the Subconscious. The Critical Faculty of the Conscious Mind heavily guards this model.

With regard to a Subconscious Illness Paradigm we recognize that there is an erroneous or incorrect perception at its base. Its underlying message was reinforced by *other incorrect perceptions* (Figure 11), and each additional incorrect perception strengthened and deepened our belief in the first one.

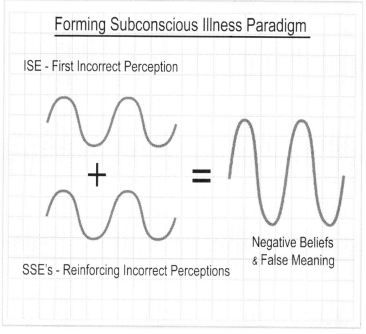

Figure 11

Here is a very common example to explain the process. Young children hear their parents argue loudly and cannot properly understand what is happening. Limited vocabulary and lack of developed critical thinking prevent them from comprehending anything about the argument. They can *only* respond to the *tone* of the verbal exchange between the parents.

As the argument continues it becomes louder. The child hears his/her name repeatedly during the argument. The child's Mind begins to *create an association* between hearing his/her name and the intense emotions of the argument. The child starts to think, feel and believe *that he/she* is the cause of the parent's unhappiness. In an attempt *to "make sense"* of the event, *the child accepts responsibility as the cause* of the argument.

As that perception sinks deeply into the Subconscious Mind, an ISE is now formed. Intuitively the child sensed it was something *he or she* did or *something about them* that caused the argument. In-turn this causes the child to feel badly. Each time this scenario repeated itself, the child's conclusion was reinforced. The Mind Patterns deepened and the belief grew stronger that the parents would be much happier if the child were not there!

The child's conclusion was *not based* on *real or meaningful knowledge* or reason for the parents' argument. *Incorrectly*, the child's conclusion was based on *a very limited perception* of what *really* transpired.

Over time the child's incorrect perception became reinforced. Now the child is three years older and hears the parents talking about how best to communicate with the child when the child misbehaves.

Each parent presents a different view. The father preaches for a harsh punishment while the mother suggests more understanding of the child. This event (discussion) becomes heated and loud once again.

One more time, the child learns that he or she is *the cause of another argument* and one once again the cause for the parent's unhappiness. It was an easy conclusion because the topic of the argument (in this case parenting) was beyond the comprehension and understanding of the child.

Here too, the child's conclusion of the event was not based on real knowledge, *but rather a limited perception*. The child did not understand the parents' perspective and could not possibly grasp the concept of adult relationships or communication between spouses. Yet the underlying message to the Subconscious was already familiar, and the ISE reinforced that *"My parents will be better off or happier if I was not here"*

The law of hypnotic compounding explains the power of repetition. It states that the first suggestion accepted by the Subconscious Mind is weak. A second suggestion reinforces and strengthens the first (weak) suggestion, the third suggestion reinforces and strengthens the second, and in-turn strengthens the first, and the suggestion becomes stronger with each repetition.

In the case of *incorrect perceptions*, repetition builds a single perception into a dominant harmful belief system. In-turn, harmful beliefs fertilize and fortify the Illness Paradigm.

Case Study: Jack - Liver Cancer

One of my clients described himself as a *"Mama's boy."* He was a skinny frail boy who preferred to play with make-believe friends rather than with trucks or to play football. I will refer to him as Jack. Jack's father wanted him to be more like a *"real"* boy. He wanted a boy that played with the other children on the block, a boy he could teach the sport of football he used to play.

Because Jack was not drawn to those activities, his dad often said things like: *"you act like a girl"*, *"stop being such a wimp,"* or *"you better stop crying like a baby, or I will give you something to really cry about. "*

Jack quickly learned that he could not live up to his dad's expectations and was a disappointment. He was not the boy his dad always wanted. His lack of "boyish" character was a major source of embarrassment and shame for his dad.

As Jack grew older, those incidents simply added fuel to an already burning fire. Each derogatory comment and negative statement was like a drop of poison administered into the veins of Jack's Subconscious Mind, a storage reservoir of pain and self-contempt.

Each negative statement compounded the one before, and without a voice of reason to contradict his dad's statements, Jack began to believe his dad would have been better off if he were never born.

Like any child, Jack wanted more than anything to please his dad, and for his dad to be proud of him. Unfortunately he was not able to accomplish that. His dad's toxic comments and suggestions, like rain drops falling into a barrel, filled it and overflowed as time went on.

Jack's Subconscious Mind responded to the overflow by forming the belief that his dad would be happier if he was not here. The Subconscious Mind is literal and will produce the conditions reflected by our beliefs. In this case, death was the ultimate way to please his dad.

At the age 27 Jack's goal achieving Subconscious Mind finally delivered a condition that reflected his belief: Jack was diagnosed with liver cancer.

Blind trust and a figure of authority is all it takes to swing the door of the Subconscious Mind wide open. There are many authority figures in our lives: parents, family, friends, teachers, popular classmates and others in whom we place our blind trust.

Love, fear, shock and confusion are just a few examples of circumstances or situations with the power to open the door of the Subconscious Mind as well.

The old proverb *"Death and life are in the power of the tongue"* tells us a great deal about the possible building blocks of the Subconscious Illness Paradigm words. Words we accept and allow in our Minds, can be transmuted into thought paradigms and then expressed in the form of success or failure, sickness or health.

Blame

It is tempting to place blame on Jack's dad or even Jack himself. However, I strongly encourage my clients not to fall into the common Mind trap of blame, judgment and guilt.

My sincere belief is that parents, caretakers, teachers and authority figures intended to do the best they could. Unfortunately, it may not have been good enough. All adults have their own Illness Paradigm, their own sets of beliefs, and their own life struggles. They might have lacked the knowledge and capacity to do better.

There is no denying that mistakes were made along the way, but focusing on blame and judgment and the pain they provoked is counterproductive to our healing. It is like holding hot coals in our hand, intending to throw them at someone, and yet we are the ones who are burned by continuing to hold them.

Blaming yourself is unfair. Our Illness Paradigm was programmed long before we knew it was even happening. Beliefs and self-concepts were developed as children, before we became rational thinking adults and before we realized that adults may be wrong.

Turning Thoughts Around

Every *first perception* is a *potential ISE*. However it is important to note that *most ISE remain dormant forever or dissolve as we grow up*. If the parents would have expressed unconditional love to the child right there and then, then the child would most likely have come to a different decision about the meaning of those events. Their meaning would be constructive rather than destructive. That did not happen, and the underlying negative message of their ISE was compounded by other events. The illness message was now running at a Subconscious level.

But all is not lost! As adults we can intervene and affect change within our Subconscious Mind *long after the Illness Paradigm was formed.* Because the integral components of the Illness Paradigm reside in the Subconscious Mind, *psychotherapy per se is insufficient.* We must use a therapeutic process such as Immersive Healing to bypass the Conscious Mind.

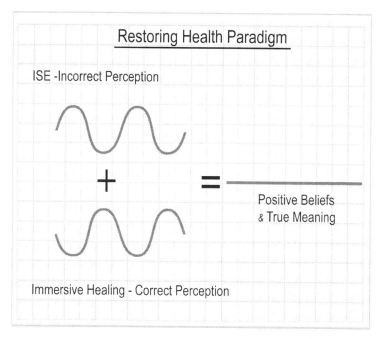

Figure 12

The Restoring Health Paradigm in Figure 12 illustrates how two opposing thought wave patterns, one positive and one negative, can cancel each other. There is *no more conflict when an incorrect perception is corrected.* Balance, comfort, health and well-being can exist along with conflict. As adults we can take charge of our own lives. In fact, it is our responsibility to care for ourselves, and thus correct our negative perceptions and consequential illness.

Chapter 6

Scientific Foundation for Immersive Healing

Immersive Healing is an evidence-based practice grounded in the scientific study of Psychoneuroimmunology (PNI). As an Immunotherapeutic approach to healing, Immersive Healing was specifically developed to revive and fortify the innate Immune System, the natural defense system of the body, by healing the non-physical aspects of cancer.

Non-physical aspects, such as harmful beliefs, erroneous perceptions and emotional conflicts, reside within the Subconscious Mind. These non-physical aspects are considered to be the root causes of illness. Healing occurs when those aspects are addressed and resolved.

These non-physical aspects of cancer *"weigh heavily"* on the Immune System and disrupt its proper functioning. According to Dr. Bruce Lipton, all energy messages influence all inter-connected cells. The non-physical aspects suppress, inhibit and directly impact the proper functioning of the Immune System. In so doing, they produce the conditions whereby illness can thrive within the body. A weak and poorly functioning Immune System needs to be revived and healed in order to combat the illness.

The Birth of Psychoneuroimmunology (PNI)

PNI is an exciting field of scientific research which examines the interaction between the psychological processes (primarily stress) and the nervous and Immune System of the human body.

PNI focuses on two related topics:

1. The relationship between the nervous system and Immune System.

2. How the mental process affects health.

While the concept of the Mind-Body connection is central in many ancient cultures, PNI has provided the scientific evidence for its mechanism. Psychoneuroimmunology includes: *"Psycho"* which refers to your thinking, emotions and mood states, *"Neuro"* which includes the neurological and neuroendocrine systems in your body, and *"Immunology"* which encompasses your cellular structures and Immune System.

PNI opens the door to a new era of Medicine, whereby people will be educated and encouraged to tap into, utilize and mobilize their innate healing resources for their own well-being.

PNI will be called upon to integrate and combine its new skills with the best science that Medicine has to offer. Knowledge of the Mind-Body interactions empowers us to make changes in the way we think and live, to better care for ourselves and properly maintain a state of health.

However, the truth remains that *all healing is still self-healing and the resources to heal reside within each of us.* Recall Mr. Wright, who had the "right stuff" within to produce recovery and healing.

In 1975, the psychologist Dr. Robert Ader and his colleague Dr. Nicholas Cohen at the University of Rochester conducted a series of experiments designed to measure the classical Pavlovian Conditioning Process. They used a combination of saccharine-laced water and the nausea-inducing drug Cytoxan to condition lab rodents to associate the sweetened water with a bad bellyache. Once successful, the rodents received the sweet water alone without the accompanying drug. The purpose of the experiment was to see how long it might take them to forget the association between the two.

According to Dr. David Felten of the University of Rochester, "Unexpectedly, during the second month, the rats began to fall prey to disease and to die off." Investigating this unforeseen result, Ader's team explored the properties of the nausea-inducing drug they had used and found that one of its side effects was as an Immune suppressant. The rodents were conditioned not only to identify sweet water with nausea, but also with an Immune shutdown. Since the process of association is a function of the Mind, the conclusion was that their minds were controlling their Immune Systems. This was a critical discovery as Felten pointed out: "The fact of the Mind-Immune System connection had been made clear. What remained was the central question of just *how* they were connected."

Pavlov's classical experiments successfully conditioned dogs to respond physically (salivation) to the stimuli of sound (ring of a bell). Ader successfully conditioned rats to respond physically (immune shutdown) to the stimuli of taste (sweetened water).

Since the 1970s, numerous studies have confirmed the relationships between the Mind, the central nervous system, and our Immune function. Using a Paradigm similar to Ader's, these studies proved that we can condition rodents not only to suppress their Immune function but also to enhance their Immune response. Through his research on mice, Ghanta proved that conditioned elevations in the activity of natural killer (NK) cells (cells that constitute a major component of the innate Immune System and play a major role in the rejection of tumors) could be attained by using the smell of camphor as the conditioned stimulus.

Recent studies reported by the immunologist Ronald Glaser and the psychologist Janice Kiecolt-Glaser of Ohio State University College of Medicine observed Immune impairment in individuals enduring chronic stress.

In one study, thirty four caregivers of Alzheimer patients were compared with thirty four control subjects. The caregivers, being under a great deal of stress, were more likely to have more severe colds than the control subjects (J.K. Kiecolt-Glaser, Psychosomatic Medicine, 53:345-62, 1991). In a prior study, Dr. Kiecolt-Glaser compared thirty-eight married women with thirty-eight separated or divorced women. Married women were found to have better Immune function than the recently separated or divorced women (Kiecolt-Glaser et al. 1987).

These studies clearly demonstrated that the reduction of stress or the enhancement of positive emotions can boost immunity. Words and/or thoughts (the Mind) can directly affect the Immune System in humans by serving as conditioned stimuli for suppressing or enhancing immune responses.

Armed with this scientific explanation, we can ask why Medicine fails to integrate PNI into mainstream cancer treatment?

Dr. Al Barrios a noted psychologist offered the following explanation: "As I see it, there were two major stumbling blocks preventing Medicine to move in that direction in the past. First there did not seem to be any rational explanation how working through the Mind, would affect an organic disease such as cancer. And secondly, Medicine has not been aware of any effective tools to deal with the psychological factors."

However, both obstacles have now been removed. First, the study of PNI by mapping the immunological mechanism provided a rational explanation for how the Mind can affect cancer. Secondly, advances in the field of Hypnotherapy provide effective methods for dealing with the Subconscious integral components comprising the Illness Paradigm.

The Science of the Mind-Body Relationship

Dr. Ader is credited with introducing the term "Psychoneuroimmunology", and his experiments provided the core clinical evidence used by others to explore the link between the Mind and Body. PNI research helps us to understand the relationship between mental and emotional states, the human nervous system and the functioning of the Immune System.

We now have a logical and rational explanation of how the Mind can affect organic or physical health. The lessons from PNI research are compelling medical researchers to reexamine old assumptions. The debate has shifted dramatically from questioning whether the Mind has any role in causing disease to *whether the Mind can influence the physical body enough for disease to develop or healing to occur.*

While more scientific research is required to provide a complete answer to this question, nowadays many notable institutions around the world are investigating the promising potential of PNI. Clearly, if Mind States have such a vital role in the origin and negative perpetuation of disease, then conversely Mind States can be utilized or mobilized to bring about positive health and well-being.

This does not mean we are without insight into the working of the Mind. Deepak Chopra M.D. says that *"Belief has a role to play in any form of therapy, whether chemotherapy, radiation, surgery or alternative Medicine."*

What is Immunotherapy?

Illness is a balancing act between disease producing agents and the body's ability to defend against these agents. A stronger Immune System means greater resilience and increased capacity to fend off potential threats.

Healing takes place naturally within the body all the time. However, healing and the body's innate healing mechanism is not entirely understood. Immunotherapy is a general term for any therapy designed to *stimulate or suppress, enhance and restore the Immune System* in people affected by disease. In conventional Medicine, immunotherapy takes the form of biological therapy or biotherapy. In integrative health care, immunotherapy utilizes Mind resources to revive the dormant Immune Response.

Immersive Healing works in the realm of the Subconscious Mind where all bodily and immune functions are governed. It offers an advanced, non-invasive and holistic methodology to healing cancer, one that utilizes an Immunotherapeutic approach.

The Immunotherapeutic method of Immersive Healing is based on three basic premises:

1. The body's natural Immune System is designed to defend against all illnesses, cancer included.
2. Harmful States of Mind (stress and hopelessness, etc.) and negative Subconscious Programming, suppress the proper functioning of the body's natural Immune System.
3. If these harmful states of Mind can be healed, the Immune System can be revived and cancer prevented or healed.

The power of the Immune System to defend and sustain the body is enormous. To explain the level of this power, think of death and what happens to the body after we die. All bodily functions stop in death, including the Immune System. Without a functioning Immune System, the body begins to decay in just a few hours after bacteria and other biological agents invade. These agents do not affect us in any way when we are alive and armed with a fortified Immune System.

The above evidence concludes that physiological changes are, in-fact, directly influenced by changes in our mental state. Therefore, by restoring the mental state to one of harmony and balance, we also restore balance to the physical body. Cancer threatens many lives, but must it remain a threat? Succumbing to the threat will make you its slave and servant in fear for your life. The important thing to understand is that you *can fight cancer* and do not need to be a slave to its fear. Other people have done it. Cancer is a serious disease, but on the other side, spending your life with this disease allows you to understand how fragile life can be.

Chapter 7

Immersive Healing for Cancer

Immersive Healing evolved as a non-invasive, holistic, adjunct approach to medical cancer treatment. It enhances the efficacy of conventional medical treatment by healing the non-physical aspects of the illness. In some cases, Immersive Healing will also reduce the amount of medical interventions needed.

Chemotherapy, radiation and surgery save lives, and it is important to acknowledge their role and function in cancer treatment. They do so however at a high cost for the patient's quality of life and well being. The current medical paradigm is fixated on cancer damage control and the treatment of cellular biology, with indifference to approaches outside that mindset.

Scientists have dreamed of using the body's own Immune defenses to fight cancer for many years. Remarkable progress has been made in gaining an understanding of how to restore the Immune System. Science harnessed medicine for that purpose as an external force to boost its function. Immersive Healing provides a new approach to mobilizing the body's Immune defenses to defeat cancer from within.

Millions of cancer patients have experienced, tolerated and survived the severe side effects and invasive nature of chemotherapy, radiation and surgery because *their will-to-live was stronger than their wish-to-die.* Cancer patients intuitively know that certain changes must be made in their lives in order to achieve different results. By continuing to think and behave in the same way, we are most likely to re-experience the same limiting and threatening conditions in our lives. Doing the same thing the same way will bring about the same results.

Unfortunately, none of the current medical treatments focus on eliminating the non-physical root cause of cancer, only its symptoms. Immersive Healing fills that void by working within the Mind to eliminate the Subconscious integral components that created the illness in the first place. By treating the root cause, there is so much to gain from every dimension and every perspective.

The medical Paradigm evolved through scientific research on the anatomical and physiological composition of the body. It separated the individual from the disease, and in so doing failed to address the root cause of the disease. For healing to take place, the person and the disease cannot and should not be separated.

The Whole Person approach to healing is not a new idea. It has been around since the beginning of modern medicine. Hippocrates (460 BC - 357 BC), the father of modern Medicine, said "It is more important to know what sort of person has a disease than to know what disease a person has." This statement resonates with each one of my clients and may resonate with you as well.

This explains the continued growth and resurrection of non-invasive therapies that can be used alongside the doctors' physical-only approach to managing their disease.

During my years of practice, I have researched many healing modalities looking for a goal-oriented therapeutic process bridging science and healing. Immersive Healing accomplishes that goal because it provides a systematic, empowering healing plan with positive and promising results. With Immersive Healing, there is no medication, no downtime, no side effects, and so much to gain by adding it to your healing plan.

Goals of Immersive Healing

The three main goals of Immersive Healing are to:

1. Heal the underlying non-physical aspects of the illness residing in the Subconscious Mind that promotes the illness from within.

2. Revive and optimize the functioning of the Immune-Response system and the natural Immune System.

3. Facilitate a continuing state of healing with the purpose of preventing secondary cancer.

People touched by cancer agree that there is more to their illness than just the tumor itself. Cancer is not an overnight event, but rather an outcome from the blossoming of seeds planted in the fertile ground of the Mind long ago. The battle with cancer is fought on many fronts, and people fighting for their lives know there is more to healing and health than only the regimens of surgery, chemotherapy or radiation.

To truly heal, we must transcend the one dimensional mindset of illness embedded in the current medical approach. We must look beyond genetics, germs, and pollutants, and address the real root cause of cancer, the unheard cry of the wounded Mind. By healing the integral Subconscious components inflaming the Mind Wound, we heal the calling of the Subconscious Mind for illness.

As the healing process unfolds, internal stressors that weigh heavily and suppress the proper functioning of the Immune System are healed. Energy previously dedicated to manage the inflamed Subconscious components can now be utilized to ignite and revive the dormant Immune Response and strengthen the body's own defense system.

Because Immersive Healing gets to the root of the deep-seated patterns of cancer, it also helps prevent cancer from resurfacing in secondary medical conditions after the primary problem is successfully addressed by surgery, radiation, chemotherapy or medication.

Hypnotherapy and Healing: Foundation and History

Dave Elman (1900–1967), considered by many as the father of modern Hypnotherapy, laid the groundwork for applying the protocols of hypnotic regression to healing. Among the many practitioners who followed Elman's teaching was Steve Parkhill, a renowned hypnotist and author of *Answer Cancer - The Healing of a Nation*. Parkhill not only filled Elman's big shoes but was also able to leap forward. He crafted, polished and advanced Elman's technique to a new level. In doing so, he created a truly unique therapeutic process that helped so many to heal from cancer and reclaim their lives.

Healing takes place naturally within the body only after the internal, unresolved emotional and mental patterns promoting illness from within are healed. Failing to heal from within, the Subconscious "that calls" for illness will continue to echo its message throughout the body, and illness will flourish again. These unresolved patterns are the mental blueprint of illness.

Immersive Healing is based on the premise that *healing of the body requires healing of the Subconscious Mind*. Immersive Healing provides a therapeutic structure and systematic process that safely allow the healing of the Mind. Doctors can see cancer cells, but they cannot see the hidden factors in the Subconscious Mind that contribute to the illness. The hidden factors must be addressed and not ignored.

Immersive Healing uses Hypnotherapy as its therapeutic vehicle to bypass the Conscious Mind and reach the Subconscious Mind. Hypnotherapy has long been an ally in the fight against cancer. Up to now, it has been mostly applied as part of a symptoms management approach to treat, nausea, fatigue or pain.

With advancements in the field of hypnosis, such as the development of Regression to Cause by Parkhill, we are now able to intervene and support the Immune System as it defends against illness.

We are now able to:

1. Identify and resolve the Subconscious integral components that promote illness from within.

2. Revive the body's innate Immune Response and strengthen one's resolve to heal.

The Difference between Immersive Healing and Psychotherapy

Psychotherapy and Immersive Healing both engage the Mind, but there are conceptual, pragmatic and systematic differences between the practices. Traditionally, *psychotherapy* tends to focus on the *intellectual understanding* of a problem by interacting with the Conscious Mind. On the other hand, *Immersive Healing* uses *Hypnotherapy* to engage the Subconscious Mind while bypassing the Conscious Mind.

Engaging with the Subconscious means recalling experiences the Conscious Mind cannot remember. The ISE and many SSE will not be discovered by conscious recollection because they are buried deep in the Subconscious Mind. Most ISEs are formed in the first few years of life, sometimes even before birth, a time completely erased from the Conscious Mind.

Another fundamental difference between Psychotherapy and Hypnotherapy is the level *of authenticity* clients can expect to achieve. This stems from working with different realms of the Mind. Hypnosis allows the client to recall and relive past experiences, to relive them in the *exact* same way they were originally experienced when they first occurred, as if they were happening in the present moment. The same feelings and emotions can be revisited to their full expression due to the capacity of the Subconscious Mind to revivify the information stored from a particular moment in time.

The client can once again experience every aspect of the event. The sounds, smells, tastes, and sights all come to life as if they were back in the time that it actually happened. Back "then" *now becomes* "right now."

During psychotherapy sessions, clients typically talk about their experiences, hence the label Talk Therapy. They use their ability to rationalize or intellectualize past experiences, to look at their experiences from the outside as an observer rather than as a participant.

This highlights another very significant difference between the two practices: the time line to affect change. Affecting change in the Subconscious Mind brings about immediate change in real time. Changes made to the Subconscious Mind result in immediate changes to the Mind, and therefore changes to the body.

Immersive Healing is a goal-oriented process, a short-term therapeutic process with a defined beginning, middle, and end. It typically requires a minimum of five sessions and a maximum of ten. I find this structure to be extremely beneficial and productive for my clients. By contrast, psychotherapy in its various forms is an ongoing and continuous therapeutic process. The success or lack thereof is measured over a long period of time, months and even years.

Perhaps the most relevant difference between Psychotherapy and Hypnotherapy is the fact that the Subconscious Mind is the part of the Mind that governs bodily functions, including Immune functions. Therefore, we must engage the Subconscious Mind in order to revive the innate Immune-Response.

Only in the Subconscious Mind will we be able to identify, address and heal all the non-physical factors inhibiting the proper function and performance of the Immune System.

The comparison between Immersive Healing and Psychotherapy is summarized in the following table.

Immersive Healing (Hypnotherapy) versus Psychotherapy Overview

Immersive Healing	Psychotherapy
Works in the realm of the Subconscious Mind (Hypnotherapy)	*Works in the realm of the Conscious Mind (talk therapy)*
Effect is internal (health, sickness)	*Effect is external (behavior, success, failure)*
Experiential (revivification of experience, authenticity stems from reliving past experiences)	*Intellectual (rationalization, analyzing, observing)*
Change is immediate in real time	*Change is incubating and takes place over time*
Short-term therapeutic process 5 – 10 sessions	*Long-term therapeutic process,*

In its natural state, the Mind and Body are in equilibrium. The Mind-Body equilibrium reveals itself as health and well-being. Immersive Healing is all about *restoring* the state of equilibrium, and in doing so, *restoring* the state of health.

Authenticity in Healing

In essence, all healing is self-healing because healing is an inner process. At the root of every healing process is the decision to be in control of the process. It is a continuing and ongoing event taking place from within.

Authenticity is the bridge that allows changes in the Mind to be expressed and felt in the body. Healing must be felt and experienced, be real and authentic in order to bring about real and lasting change.

Authenticity is the key factor that makes Hypnotherapy and Immersive Healing so effective. Authenticity is the byproduct of a state of complete immersion and absorption, or the *hypnotic state*.

The United States Department of Education defines hypnosis as *"The bypass of the Critical Factor of the Conscious Mind (one's ability to critique, reason and judge) and the establishment of acceptable selective thinking."*

Critical Faculty

Critical Faculty refers to the ability of the Conscious Mind to analyze input from the five senses: touch, taste smell, sight and hearing. We explored this at length in the discussion of the Human Mind Model in Chapter 4. Within this context, it may be helpful to think of the Critical Faculty as a safety mechanism designed to protect the information stored within the Subconscious Mind. To experience the Critical Factor at work, consider the following math: does $1 + 1 = 7$? *Of course not!*

The Critical Faculty of the Conscious Mind rejects $1 + 1 = 7$ and any other wrong answer because it does not match the existing perception and knowledge that it has stored.

The Critical Faculty regarding our perceptions about ourselves works in a similar way. Think for a moment of how you respond to praise and compliments. For example, when someone says "you are so talented" or "you are so beautiful," does the little inner-voice say "of course I am", or does it say "no I am not"? The point is, if the compliment contradicts your perception of self, it will be rejected.

In order to facilitate the hypnotic state for Immersive Healing, we must bypass this safety mechanism. Otherwise, access to the realm of the Subconscious Mind will be denied. When successful, access to the Subconscious Mind is attained and clients are able to recall, relive and heal the Subconscious Illness Paradigm.

The Subconscious Illness Paradigm is the collective name for all the *integral components and non-physical aspects of illness residing in the Subconscious Mind*. It refers to erroneous perceptions, distorted self-views, harmful belief systems, etc.

Authenticity is an outcome. It is the result of working in the realm of the emotional Subconscious Mind. It is like the experience of reading a book when you become fully absorbed and identify with the personality and emotions of the characters. You share their feelings as if you are walking in their shoes or listening to their mental intimate inner dialog.

Have you ever become so deeply involved with a character in a story that it felt real and authentic? This is especially true when telling the story of your own life. You have firsthand participation in everything the main character experiences in this story because the main character is you!

This deep level of immersion is established during hypnosis. It helps reduce Mind noise and increase authenticity. Mind noise, such as automatic and intrusive thoughts, negative mental images and stressors, can inhibit complete immersion, and therefore inhibit the natural ongoing process of healing.

This supreme level of authenticity is used in Immersive Healing for complete revivification of past events. Revivification of past events permits the recall of specific conditions and circumstances where the seed planting of the Subconscious Illness Paradigm is stored.

Immersive Healing employs revivification of the event, while traditional forms of psychotherapy rely on the client's conscious ability to remember and recall past events, their details, feelings and emotions.

Here the client authentically recalls the whole event, intact with the feelings and emotions originally felt and experienced when it first happened. It is like stepping into a still frame picture that becomes a video of this moment in time. You actively participate rather than only look at it.

Ultimately authenticity permits transmutation of erroneous and harmful perceptions into correct and positive ones. Updated and corrected perceptions of past events lead to healing of the Subconscious Illness Paradigm and ultimately the healing of the physical body.

Revivification versus Remembering

The most important key to successful therapy and real transformation is revivification. Some people have the gift of sight: they can close their eyes and vividly and literally recall images in their Mind's eye. In my experience, those people are the exception and not the rule.

The great majority of people use a combination of mental vision, thoughts and imagination, much like daydreaming, to breathe life into their experiences.

To consciously remember what happened (as in memories) is altogether different from a revivification of the experience. Memory is often flat or one-dimensional, and for the most part fleeting. Furthermore, memories from early childhood tend to be partial and incomplete. On the other hand, by reliving the same childhood experience, one has access to actual thoughts as they occurred at that moment in time. Reviving that experience replays the actual feelings as they felt at that time.

Engaging the Conscious Mind means being the observer of our own process. It means we are limited in our ability to enforce change. Change on the conscious level may be attainable over a long period, but time may be a luxury that someone with cancer cannot afford.

Reliving an experience, we become active participants in it, and this means change can and does happen in real time. The key to a successful transformation is that it must *feel real and, therefore, believable.*

Immersive Healing provides a clear and more realistic understanding of past events where the seed of illness is found. Such events are considered as the point of origin of the illness or Initial Sensitizing Event (ISE). When adult clients regress and relive events from an early period of life, they can utilize mental, emotional and spiritual resources that the child, they once were, did not have.

Processing the same event through the Mind of the grown-up adult rather than a child, they are bound to arrive at a different decision about the meaning of a specific event that occurred in their lives. This in turn allows them to change the way they feel and to shift their perception of the event from negative, harmful and painful, to positive and helpful.

Immersed in the hypnotic state, the client gets to explore and discover beneficial outcomes previously hidden in past events. It is a freeing process that cultivates wisdom and leads to insights and realizations about life.

When added to the accumulated authentic experience, this wisdom is used to dissolve the current Subconscious Illness Paradigm and prevent it from forming again.

The Hypnotic Protocol of Regression to Cause

The value in revisiting the ISE is the ability to re-perceive it correctly instead of incorrectly. If an incorrect perception led to a distorted or false meaning and harmful beliefs, then correct perceptions will lead to true meanings and positive beliefs.

Positive beliefs and correct perceptions are the *seeds of the Health Paradigm*, and harmful beliefs, and erroneous perception are the *seeds of the Illness Paradigm*.

Regression to Cause (RTC) is a therapeutic protocol designed to uncover a perception that led to an intense emotional response within the ISE. This is not surprising because we respond emotionally to external events. The more severe our experience, the more emotional is our response to it.

RTC allows us to revive and excite the emotions surrounding the ISE for the purpose of re-examination. Reprocessing the same old information that birthed the ISE but with the skills, abilities and resources of the adult, clients arrive at a different decision about the meaning of their experience.

By changing the meaning of the ISE, it cuts-off and dissolves the Illness Paradigm from its source so that health can then be restored.

The ISE, the seed planting of the Subconscious Illness Paradigm, took place years ago. However, in the realm of the Subconscious, time is not a factor. This means that the dimension of time does not apply in the same sense measured in seconds, minutes and hours.

We often experience time distortion when we watch a movie or become immersed in any activity that requires our full and undivided attention. Then "time flies," as we say. In the context of RTC and healing, this suggests that events from many years ago are just as accessible and available for recall and review as events from last week.

Furthermore, the Subconscious Mind is literal: it does not know the difference between what is really experienced and what it imagined. This is why your mouth watered when you performed the Taste the Lemon exercise.

The Subconscious Mind believes its own experiences. It believes that certain past events are tied into one's condition/illness and, more specifically, it believes that the ISE is its root cause.

Belief initiates authenticity. Authenticity, is the bridge to real and lasting transformation. First is the transformation of the quality of perceptions, and then the quality of our beliefs. When the quality of our perception changes from incorrect to correct and from destructive to constructive, it leads to changes in the quality of our belief systems. Harmful and limiting beliefs become inspiring and healthy beliefs. Such changes affect the human body.

Mental Time Travel – A Scientific Fact

Physical laws do not restrict the Mind to its ethereal state of existence. It can therefore travel back in time, along the timeline of our life for healing. A timeline is a way of viewing life and life's events in a linear fashion, in chronological order from birth until death. The ability to mentally access past events and relive them in a real and authentic way is the foundation of RTC. It allows us to topple the inverted pyramid of illness and limiting symptoms by "taking" out the single can (ISE) upon which it stands (Figure 8). Now health can be resorted.

Researchers at the University of Pennsylvania provided the first neurobiological evidence of the ability of the Mind to regress. The study scientifically documented and demonstrated the ability of the mind to regress to an earlier event with a detailed account of that experience. It was concluded that the Mind possesses the ability to retrieve past events in their earliest context and use them as part of its present context. ,

Psychologists refer to this as Episodic Memory, the ability to capture detailed information of particular life events and retrieve the details years later in their full contextual form. Think of *your first kiss* or the first time you realized you were riding a bicycle on your own with no support.

During Episodic Memory, we can recall not only the features of a particular event, but everything associated with the event. The ability to reinstate the contextual information about each event is the foundation of Regression Therapy. This scientific validation is important to Regression Therapy because it increases our belief in the possibility of regression therapy. Instead of just taking a leap of *faith* and hoping to get some results, we can fully rely on the *facts* and trust we will get results.

But our ability to use "mental time travel" consciously is limited because there are only so many events on the magnitude of *the first kiss*. While such an epic event can be recalled in great details within the Conscious Mind, most life events seem unimportant, ordinary and unexciting. By utilizing the hypnotic protocol of Regression to Cause, Immersive Healing intentionally harnesses the Subconscious' ability to "travel" through our mental timeline and vividly recall events for the purpose of healing.

Cancer Stages and Immersive Healing

There are multiple staging systems for cancer. Each system is specific to a particular cancer (breast cancer, lung cancer, etc.). The most familiar system ranks cancers into five progressive stages: 0, I, II, III, and IV. Each stage provides your medical doctor with information about your condition. Each has a different treatment plan and prognosis.

The cancer staging system is used differently within the context of Immersive Healing. Each stage communicates different levels of urgency, i.e., of how often sessions need to be scheduled, the length of the sessions and other related information. Each stage can provide information about the client's state of Mind and potential emotional stress. Regardless of your cancer stage, the goals and systematic approach of Immersive Healing remain the same. The premise that *healing the cause leads to healing of the effect* is valid throughout the process.

Immersive Healing aims to help clients heal on all levels: the physical, emotional and Mind. After completing five mandatory sessions, clients may choose to focus more on the quality of life instead of healing the remnants of the Subconscious Illness Paradigm. Sometimes this is the case for people in the very late stage of cancer. Overall, my clients know that there is always hope for healing. Despite diagnoses of stage IV cancer, many of them push forward and continue to fight for their health and well-being.

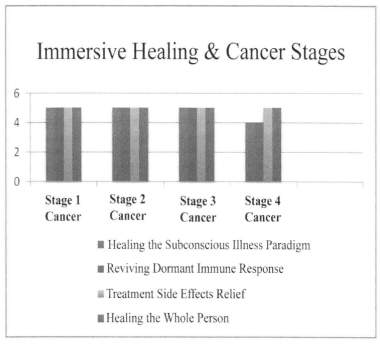

Figure 13

Immersive Healing and Chemotherapy

Chemotherapy remains one of the "three" main treatments of cancer. While researchers continue to seek more gentle treatment, current chemotherapy treatment usually has adverse physical side effects including nausea, vomiting, hair loss etc.'. It also has emotional side effects such as anticipatory anxiety and fear.

Immersive Healing utilizes the power of Hypnotherapy to increase the client's comfort level before, during and after medical treatment. It accomplishes this by reducing a patient's psychological distress, alleviating fear and anticipatory nausea.

Immersive Healing also helps clients change their attitude about chemotherapy as difficult, painful and frightening to positive and healing. This shift in perception enhances the body's ability to tolerate the drugs administered, and thereby help people maintain a higher quality of life. People viewing the procedure as health-supporting rather health-damaging can more easily sustain their sense of well-being.

Immersive Healing can further provide clients with tools for self-help and self-care. This is especially valuable when physical discomfort or pain is a side effect. Clients learn how to reduce and desensitize those sensations themselves.

Essentially, desensitizing discomfort need only be practiced with the expressed advice from your doctor. This way, you avoid reducing important physical sensations that convey information about events taking place in the body. It is important for patients to communicate any change in physical or emotional experience to their doctor for proper diagnosis and care.

Immersive Healing and Surgery

The very thought of surgery produces anxieties, and fear and worry consume our attention. Apart from worrying about potential complications, surgery, even "minor" surgery, involves risk and requires recovery time.

As an elective therapeutic process, Immersive Healing offers clients the opportunity to become active participants in their own healing process. This makes them feel more in control of their lives.

Clients can transform feelings such as stress, anxiety, hopelessness and fear into hope and empowerment. This sense of empowerment has tremendous value as it translates into a strong will-to-live.

As reported by many studies, patients who suffered from high levels of stress required more sedation and anesthesia during surgery. They also experienced more postoperative pain and needed more time to recover.

To mitigate the effect of stress on patients and help prepare them for surgery, researchers have suggested a short intervention with hypnosis. In one particular experiment with a group of breast cancer patients, researchers found women who received hypnosis intervention before surgery did far better than the control group that did not undergo hypnosis.

In a study reported by Montgomery et al in the Journal of the National Cancer Institute in 2007, patients who were hypnotized briefly before breast cancer surgery needed fewer anesthetics and had less pain, nausea and fatigue after the procedure. The benefits extended to the health care system with substantial cost savings mainly because of reduced time of surgery.

According to Guy Montgomery, director of Mount Sinai School of Medicine's Integrative Behavioral Medicine Program and lead author of the study: "The vast majority of patients can have some benefit from doing this.   To me it's a no-brainer: It helps patients, and it saves money."

We tend to stress out and worry either because we perceive a situation to be dangerous, difficult, or painful, or because we do not believe we have the resources to cope. The first point is about perception and the second about belief. Immersive Healing offers relief on both fronts. Firstly, it helps the client change their perception of the surgery from a dangerous, difficult or painful event to a safe and swift procedure practiced day in and day out by highly skilled professionals. Secondly, it strengthens the client's belief and confidence in their inner resources as well as the ability to cope and heal from surgery.

Understandably, surgery is viewed by our Mind as a threat. It is an invasive procedure designed to produce changes to our body. Remember, one of the primary functions of the Mind is to protect and ensure we are safe and secure.

By changing the client's perception, enhancing belief in their own inner resources and instilling a positive mental expectancy about treatment outcome, Immersive Healing lessens fear and anticipatory anxiety. This has a positive effect on the surgical procedure. Ultimately, Immersive Healing helps patients to maintain a high quality of life.

Dr. Michael Schmitz, director of pediatric pain Medicine at Arkansas Children's Hospital in Little Rock, described the state of anesthesia as consisting of four basic conditions: amnesia or loss of memory, analgesia or pain relief, sedation and relaxation. "Hypnosis is used to assist with the other parts of anesthesia not covered by the local anesthetic," said Schmitz, explaining that it can help patients enter a calm, relaxed state, during which discomfort is tolerable and quickly forgotten.

Immersive Healing and Radiation

Radiation is a localized event, unlike chemotherapy that takes place throughout the whole body. It can destroy cancer cells, control the growth of cancer and help improve the symptoms. But the invasive nature of radiation has *substantial psychological distress* that can inhibit its effectiveness and impact the patient's quality of life.

Side effects from radiation are both *physiological and emotional*. Physiological side effects include nausea, pain, blood pressure, skin problems, hair loss and many others. Emotional side effects include anticipatory anxiety, sadness, hostility, tension, fatigue, confusion and overall mood.

Depending on the type and dose, radiation side effects may vary widely in their severity. The occurrence of side effects or their severity can cause patients to *skip, miss or discontinue* medical treatment. The American Cancer Society estimates that 50% of cancer patients *do not* follow through and complete their full treatments.

Disturbance to the patient's daily routine can also influence the severity of side effects. This fosters a feeling of helplessness as if they have lost control over the illness. Immersive Healing helps to reduce the severity of some physical side effects and improve the client's comfort level during radiation treatment. Patients enjoy a higher rate of success if they enter treatment with the right frame of Mind.

My clients report feeling empowered when provided with the opportunity to actively participate in their own healing process. The internal sense of *"being in control"* helps them maintain autonomy and avoid falling into the common negative *Mind-Traps*. Feeling more in control and active participation in your healing process can help avoid becoming a medical statistic.

Chapter 8

Immersive Healing: Step by Step

Immersive Healing is a systemic therapeutic process. Success of Immersive Healing depends on our ability to complete the entire process according to a structured protocol. Each session begins with hypnotic induction to *bypass of the* Critical Faculty of the Conscious Mind. It focuses the client's attention, heightens expectations and beliefs about a desired outcome, and ensures that the client becomes absorbed and immersed in their inner experience.

According to The Human Mind Model (Figure 3), the Critical Faculty refers to the capacity of the Conscious Mind to reason, make judgments, rationalize, intellectualize, and accept or reject information. Once the Critical Faculty is bypassed, the client is in the hypnotic state providing access to the Subconscious Mind.

Immersive Healing follows the same logical process to heal Mind Wounds as to heal physical wounds.

Step-by-Step Process for Treating Physical Wounds:

Step one:
Identify the location of the physical wound in the body.

Step two:
Examine and clean the wound.

Step three:
Apply the antiseptic to promote healing and protect it from infection.

Step four:
Apply a bandage that will protect it from the elements.

Step five:
The wound needs time to heal.

Step-by-Step Process to Heal Mind Wounds

Step one:
Locate the Initial Sensitizing Event (ISE), the origin of the Illness Paradigm.

Step two:
Clean the ISE by releasing the intense emotions buried deep inside.

Step three:
Change an incorrect perception to a correct perception. The erroneous perception that gave birth to the illness must be changed, and a new corrected perception must be put in place so that the healing process can begin. It's like changing the chemistry of the physical wound with an antiseptic balm

Step four:
Forgiveness must be applied to the Mind Wound. Forgiveness acts as the bandage. Forgiving and forgiveness anchor the new correct perception in consciousness.

Step five:
The last step in the healing process is to assimilate it into our awareness.

Step 1: Regression to ISE

To better understand how each step in Immersive Healing works to heal cancer, we need to revisit Steve Parkhill's inverted pyramid (Figure 8)

The conventional medical approach to saving lives is that *when a cancer tumor can be removed it should be removed.* This is certainly necessary because removing the tumor often buys precious and necessary time for patients.

But there is a *Catch 22* to only removing the cancer cells. Treating *only* the physical wound (the cancer) and ignoring the associated Mind Patterns leaves the same Subconscious Illness Paradigm that created the illness in the Subconscious Mind. If we leave the Subconscious Illness Paradigm (SIP) unchanged, intact and in place, the *Subconscious Mind will find another place to manifest the illness.* It may appear in another organ or in a different part of the body.

The root origin still exists, and until it is removed the Subconscious Mind will find another means to express itself. The non-physical root origin of the cancer *will not go away just because the cancer cells are cut, poisoned or removed.* We cannot see or touch it like we can the cancer. The complex nature of the Subconscious Minds relationship to illness is treated affectively with Immersive Healing.

Medical protocols numb cancer symptoms. They cut it, burn it, poison it or remove it! Doctors have the power to mute the symptom, *but they cannot mute the message the Subconscious sends to the physical body.* That message will continue to echo through the nervous system, and in many cases will result in secondary cancer. Unfortunately, this is the most neglected phase of healing. Conventional cancer treatment does little to prevent cells from regrouping, proliferating, and forming new tumors.

It is very important to understand that physical *symptoms are the tangible evidence of what is going on in your Subconscious Mind.* If ignored and unattended, the Subconscious Mind *must and will* find another way to get its *message* of illness out into the body and that its *deeper intimate needs are not being met.* Perhaps it is this message that prompts us to seek psychotherapy in the first place. After all, *"intellect"* is the main tool we use to navigate our way through life's decisions.

Psychology is immensely valuable for many purposes. However, in the context of illness, its value is in treating and healing *only* the level of SSE and *not* the ISE.

Based on the Human Mind Model, the Critical Faculty of the Conscious Mind *will reject* all conscious suggestions that are not in harmony with what is already stored within the Subconscious Mind. The powerful human intellect is inadequate to handle a process influenced by Subconscious currents.

Bypassing the Critical Faculty of the Conscious Mind we gain access to the Subconscious Mind. The SM is where our perceptions, beliefs, concepts and values reside. When you arrive you will have knocked on the door of where the root cause of the illness originated.

When erroneous perceptions form harmful beliefs, they prompt the Subconscious Mind to call for illness. Healing can occur naturally only after those erroneous perceptions and harmful beliefs are addressed. Making changes in biology or at any other level is not enough. Change must be made at the root level of the symptom in the Subconscious Mind.

At last you can repair those *"erroneous perceptions"* and heal the non-physical aspects composing the Subconscious Illness Paradigm. With Immersive Healing, they can be healed at the very level they function. Without the reasoning power of the Conscious Mind, the literal

Subconscious Mind will then be *perfectly at peace* with any changes.

During the treatment, the Subconscious Mind is instructed to identify a specific moment in time, a situation or event *it* believes to be the ISE. The ISE is that moment when the specific perception of that event was forever altered from positive to negative.

More than one attempt may be needed to reach the ISE. In such cases, we arrive first at a Subsequent Sensitizing Event (SSE's). An SSE is a secondary life event that compounded and reinforced the original incorrect or erroneous perception of the ISE. Recalling the SSE and the ISE marks the entry to the Immersive Healing process.

Look at the image of inverted cans once again (Figure 8). Obviously removing the single can from the bottom (the ISE), causes the whole structure to collapse and fall down.

This model of the ISE represents a universal truth of nature. Every tree began life as a single seed just as every illness symptom has a Subconscious seed in the form of the ISE. As the tree seed germinates it grow into a stem, shaft, branches and leaves. The tree grows from one initial seed. As the Subconscious seed grows, it geminates the conditions for illness.

You can prune a tree branch, but the tree will grow similar branches usually in a different location. The practical way to stop a tree from growing is to completely remove its roots from the ground. In the case of illness, it means to identify and heal its ISE and SSE.

Step 2: Release of Emotions Buried in the ISE

Children's fairy tales often celebrate the *"happily ever after"* story ending. Of course reality is very different from a fairy tale. Even If you had a "perfect" childhood, "perfect" parents or "perfect" caretakers, life is never perfect all the time. There are moments you felt anger, pain, hurt, resentment, etc., and at some point life was less than perfect.

Everyone we ever knew - family and friends, those we love, those we dislike - left their mark on us. Their mark is with us all the time whether we are aware of it or not.

Those feelings are still very much within us, alive if not exhausted (back there and then), and they still influence our moment to moment experiences. In the reality of the Subconscious Mind, feelings are associated with specific events. Those feelings can be revived and excited for facilitating their release.

The Mind is shrouded in the fog of emotional intensity when we feel angry, afraid and resentful, making it difficult to think clearly and see things in their true perspective. Nevertheless, we have to attain mental clarity in order to properly *re-perceive and dissolve the ISE*. Think of it as a wound, a wound we must first clean to remove any debris that might inflame or infect it again.

Releasing the emotional intensity buried in the ISE results in mental clarity to perceive the event in a different and more positive way.

When the emotional fog and turmoil have been removed from our Mind, we are able to see the silver lining around the dark cloud. As Steve Parkhill said so well, *"One is able to find the good in the experience previously perceived as bad."* This ability is vital to a successful transmutation of the Illness Paradigm into a Health Paradigm.

Step 3: Changing Perception of the ISE

True and lasting healing begins from within. In fact, *all healing begins within*. Healing the Subconscious Illness Paradigm is a prerequisite to healing any physical illness. The harmful message of the Subconscious Illness Paradigm (SIP) must first be dissolved before a new one can take its place. We must also change our perception of the ISE from negative to positive.

When it comes to human perception, here is what we must consider:

1. In truth, our experience is a physical event that stems from our emotional state.

2. We assign meaning to our experiences.

3. Our choice of feeling (either negative or positive) has consequences. Our state of Mind and emotional state generate a road map both for the environment within our physical body and for our behavior.

The often repeated phrase *"we cannot change the past, we can only change the future"* is only partially true. We cannot change the facts about our past, but we can change the way we perceive them. This is because life events do not have meaning, they only have consequences.

A friend once said: *"Things can matter to me, but their meaning is up to me."*

Each person assigns their own meaning to their experiences. Only we can assign that meaning. We assign meaning to each experience in order for it to make sense to us within the context of the world we live in.

If another person has the identical experience and observed the very same event, they would undoubtedly interpret the event differently and, therefore, assign a different meaning to it.

The outcome of this necessary realization is freedom from attachment to past perceptions and beliefs. We can free ourselves from negative perceptions and harmful beliefs as soon as we realize this is true. We become free from the prison that chained us to the past perception.

"You had better eat all the food on your plate, because there are starving children in".... (*The relevant country of the day)!* If you are like me, you probably heard this statement more than once as a child.

Although this statement is more relevant to *one's patterns of behavior* rather *one's state of health*, it is a familiar one and serves a specific purpose.

As children, we did not understand the real meaning. As adults, we get it and we understand! The adult was trying to instill an appreciation for our abundance of food. Do not waste your food, respect that you have food because in many places around the world children do not have food and would love to have what you leave on your plate.

As adults, we know not everyone is fortunate to have such abundance. We want our children to understand and appreciate it as well (*if only as a motivation to eat*).

Most children do not and cannot understand the meaning of the statement, and inevitably *conclude a wrong meaning.* Unless the child has traveled across the world, the concept of life in another country or knowledge of what it is really like in another country without an abundance of food is a concept of thinking beyond their grasp. Furthermore, children who always had food cannot possibly understand the concept of hunger. The word "hunger" is far outside their thought Paradigm.

Children all too often arrive at this conclusion: If I finish all the food on my plate, my parent (or caretaker) will be pleased, happy, and they will love me more.

It is important to understand that our behavior is driven by our thoughts. As Tony Robbins said: "Everything we do in life is to either get more love or compensate for the lack of love."

The Mind's primary job is to protect us! It makes sure we feel safe and secure, and love is often synonymous with safety and security.

The message the child hears, reinforced over time, is the main reason why so many people struggle with their food habits. If you ever need a testimonial to the power of thought to affect behavior, the result of this eating pattern is weight gain accompanied by feeling out of control and its associated health problems.

Immersive Healing is unique because it allows a false or negative distortion of perception to be corrected. It lets us change the perception by allowing the adult client to go *"back in time"* in the Mind's eye and revisit that specific event and revise its meaning.

Once "there" the adult can reconnect with the child they were at the time of the specific event. Through an exchange and dialog of words (either silently or out loud), the adult helps the child to perceive the event anew with insight and wisdom. We have the capacity and ability to empower and enlighten the child to view the event as an adult.

Now the child is empowered with the perspective and reasoning power which were not there when the event was first experienced. The adult can now relive the event about cleaning the plate and arrive at its correct meaning.

Do you remember Frankl's illustration of the cylinder's projection back in Figure 1? Now this image can help to explain how Immersive Healing *can be used to change our perceptions* of events. A single event (cylinder) can have more than one meaning. From one perspective we see a circle, and from another we see a rectangle.

To discover hidden aspects and learn more about this event, we need to view it from different angles by casting the light in a different direction. (*A child's perception versus an adult's perception of the event.*) We will see the event differently, see more of "it" and be able to reach a different conclusion about the meaning of the event.

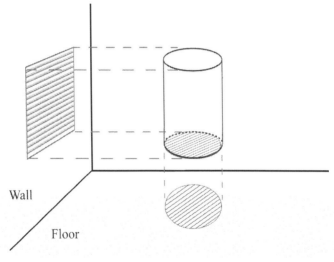

Wall

Floor

Figure 1

This new perception leads to new meaning. It brings a *change in meaning* to the original stored event and inevitably a change in behavior. At the very moment the child realizes the *true meaning* of the statement, they unlearn the original perceived meaning.... *that parental love was dependent on their action of food consumption.* At that moment, the embedded negative association shifts from *negative to neutral* (Figure 14). The original meaning ceases to be relevant and dissolves.

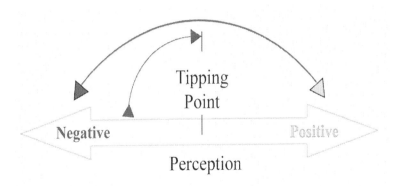

Figure 14

Once the cobwebs of the *old negative association* have been cleared, a new and more positive perspective of the event takes its place. The process must continue because there is no vacuum or void in the realm of the Mind. We must ensure that the *Pendulum of Perception (PP)* swings all the way to the positive spectrum (Figure 15).

In Immersive Healing, the Pendulum of Perception (PP) will swing to the end of the positive spectrum when the client discovers a new and positive meaning in their experience. Immersive Healing will lead the client to discover a *positive aspect or benefit previously hidden from conscious view.*

We did not and could not control our experiences as children. We perceived ourselves as victims and forged our self-image accordingly. Revisiting those early life events and rediscovering their positive and beneficial aspects provided the insight and wisdom for us to rid ourselves of the victim's outdated and false perception.

Our perception of specific events can be changed by discovering aspects previously hidden from conscious view. For healing to take place, we must look for and discover positive attributes, deeper meaning and personal outcomes that prove we have gained something worthwhile from an event we labeled as worthless.

At this stage we are free. Immersive Healing is a freeing process. We are back in control of our life and, ultimately, our destiny. Immersive Healing brings a new meaning to the phrase... "You *control your own destiny.*"

Sometimes there is *more than one positive aspect hidden from conscious perception.* The child will come to realize that their parents had perfectly good intentions in wanting them to eat properly and be healthy. They will now realize they were truly cared for and loved.

This in turn can enhance and boost self-esteem and self-image. It will improve the *child-parent relationship.* In addition, the client will develop a level of awareness so they can avoid repeating the same mistakes with their own children.

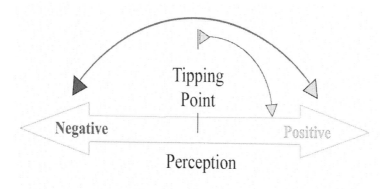

Figure 15

Through this example, we learn that *no one situation is entirely good or bad, positive or negative.* Rather, we apply meaning, perception and labels to our experiences, one way or another.

If human perception was based on *actual absolute truth,* Immersive Healing would not be necessary. Instead, it rests in the knowledge that perception is *perfectly imperfect.*

There is no perfect situation in life, at least not through human eyes. Changing perceptions allow those who survived atrocities and horror to find new meaning in their experiences. Those experiences can now have a purpose to help summon the courage to live.

We believe that *"around every dark cloud there is a silver lining."* For every bad situation there is an element of good, and we can derive *some* benefit *from every bad thing* that happens to us.

It is the discovery of *hidden meaning* that completes our *"life lesson"* stored in a particular past event. This discovery ensures that we can move on and further heal.

Step 4: Forgiveness: Healing of Erroneous Anger and Guilt

At this point in this step by step process, we have:

1. successfully identified our ISE,
2. released its emotional intensity for the purpose of clarity and,
3. changed our perception of events from negative to positive (but *not the perception of* ourselves... at least not *yet).*

Anger, criticism and other unpleasant emotions arise when we learn that our life experience is based on incorrect perceptions or influenced by our incorrect perceptions (*limitations and conditions*).

This realization lives as an *aftertaste* of guilt. Guilt is mostly toxic! I say this because feeling guilty is appropriate when we deliberately hurt or harm others or ourselves. Not feeling guilt is inhuman. Sociopaths have no sense of guilt!

Toxic guilt is the product of self-judgment. It is an erroneous thought process about doing something wrong when, in-fact, there is *no actual wrongdoing.*

Of course we prefer to blame others for our misfortunes. Blaming is much easier than taking ownership or responsibility for our lives. But unbeknownst to others, *we do not let ourselves off the hook.* In the privacy of our own Mind, we hold ourselves and no one else accountable.

Toxic guilt is the last lifeline of the Subconscious Illness Paradigm. If not forgiven and dissolved, it may recreate the conditions for illness to thrive over time.   So it is immensely important to forgive any remnant and form of toxic guilt, be it resentment, self-blame, self-pity, self-hatred or shame.

Webster's New World Dictionary defines *"to forgive"* as "to give up resentment against or the desire to punish; to excuse." For the meaning of "to excuse," we find "to release from an obligation; to permit to leave; to liberate."

In therapy, forgiveness is regarded as a central and necessary part of emotional healing. Stripped of its religious connotation, forgiveness is a therapeutic tool that we can use to transform and heal our perceptions and beliefs.

As the last piece of the healing puzzle, forgiveness is analogous to applying balm to a physical wound. It is both antiseptic and healing. Forgiveness must be understood in order to release or liberate the chains of the Subconscious Illness Paradigm.

There are many misconceptions and myths about forgiveness. It is a difficult concept for many people. Very common misconceptions are that *"one must forget in order to forgive"* and that *"forgiveness is condoning."* These misconceptions add to why we may believe it is difficult to forgive.

But forgiveness is not a form of denial, and therefore it does not require *forgetfulness*. Forgiveness is very much about remembering, but remembering what happened in a *meaningful way*. Forgiveness does not mean condoning of any action, but rather understanding what happened within the correct context.

The first step in forgiveness is to acknowledge that we do most of the suffering. Once we accept this truth, we can finally begin to free ourselves from the grip of negativity and start to exchange despair for hope. Then we can begin to create the life we want and deserve, a life free from the physical, mental, and emotional side-effects of guilt, anger, fear, etc.

Bob Brenner, a noted hypnotist, used the following analogy to clarify this statement. He asks his clients if they had ever walked down the street and happened to notice an empty soda can kicked it while walking along. He asked them why they kicked the can. Why did they do it? Did the can provoke them in any way? Did it do anything to deserve to be kicked? The answer of course is *NO. The can was simply in their path.* It is likely we have all done something similar, whether it was a soda can, a stick, a rock or anything else.

This analogy helps anyone who believes someone has *"done them wrong"* or *"kicked"* them to see the truth. The person that *"kicked"* did so not because of what we did or did not do, rather because of a feeling inside, a feeling that was there long before we crossed their path. The person who "kicked" did so because of an inner feeling, a feeling that existed long before we crossed their path and not because of what we did or did not do.

In this sense, forgiveness is a choice! Forgiving is *our choice,* to see things in their true perspective. To realize that something did in-fact happen, but its meaning is up to us. We ultimately must forgive ourselves for perceiving things that led us to feel anger, fear, resentment, shame and guilt.

Holding on to harmful feelings is like playing a tug-of-war with the Illness Paradigm. The Subconscious Mind holds one end of the rope with *the harmful past perceptions and beliefs*, and we (*consciously*) hold the other end.

All we need to do to get rid of them is let go of the rope! As soon as we let go and release our end of the rope, there is no more tension, nothing to hold on to, and so we experience freedom. This is exactly what happens when we choose to forgive. All forgiveness is, in essence, *self-forgiveness.*

Step 5: Assimilating into Present Awareness

The protocol of Hypnotic Regression to Cause is unique because it allows us to work in the past and heal different aspects of it *in the present.* Throughout the process, we get to relive and re-perceive our life in a more meaningful way. We can strengthen the child within, and grow stronger and wiser. But for the healing to be complete we must press on. First, we must test the work by aggravating painful aspects related to the client's ISE. Secondly, we must bring forth the accumulated healing and wisdom into present time awareness. This will not only ensure proper healing to the body, but also eliminate e the root cause of our cancer so it will not resurface.

In a sense, Regression Therapy is a process of deconstruction. We deconstruct the past in a way that allows us to address specific parts and elements of it. As we begin to move forward along our mental time line, we get to reconstruct our self-concept, and in doing so restore our health.

It is important for the client to have evidence of the effectiveness by moving forward through some of their SSEs. As they come across events previously registered as painful or negative in any way, they get to test their feelings about them. There is tremendous value in doing so, and the proof at hand reinforces the changes already made.

We can re-perceive past events differently and repair our perception because the adult client was able to connect with the inner child. Using the same approach, the inner child now heals and transfers all those feelings and sensations to the adult.

It is often an emotional moment when the adult client realizes that the connection with the inner child is real. It is real because the adult client feels exactly what the child feels and experiences, the same associated sensations. It is quite common for clients to say they feel bathed in warmth and light.

At this point in the treatment, we have all the pieces in place. Once again we utilize the *goal achieving capacity* of the Subconscious Mind to affect even more healing. It is just as easy for the Subconscious Mind to work into the future as it is to regress back in time.

The level of authenticity resulting from hypnotic immersion allows the client to fully experience the future. Clients will see themselves completely healed and whole. They can construct a mental road map for their Subconscious Mind to follow.

Chapter 9

Case Study: Michelle - Breast Cancer

I now present a case study to illustrate the Immersive Healing process described in the previous chapter. The client in this case study is Michelle, a 37 year old woman with stage III breast cancer. She was referred to me by her oncologist who was treating her with chemotherapy. .

A graphical illustration of the Immersive Healing process for Michele is shown in Figure 16. This figure includes all five steps involved over a period of time.

Michelle's Time Line

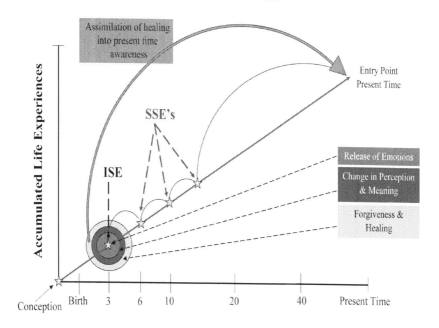

ISE: Initial Sensitizing Event

SSE: Subsequent Sensitizing Event

During her Immersive Healing treatment, Michelle successfully arrived at three different SSE's before she got to the ISE. Her time line for these events is included in Figure 16. The underlying theme of her SSE's was self-hate, shame and guilt. Each SSE represented those feelings in a different way.

For the purpose of this discussion, we will explore her SSE's from the present time backwards. Her most recent SSE (age 17) regarded an unplanned pregnancy and abortion. She was influenced to terminate the pregnancy, although she really wanted to keep the child. This open wound inflamed and compounded existing perceptions.

An earlier SSE (age 11) regarded a very poor report card from school. She recalled her mother's disappointment. Her mother made a point of saying how she had sacrificed so much just to provide for her daughter's education, insinuating that Michelle's poor performance in school was causing her mother much pain, disappointment and sorrow.

Michelle's first SSE (age 6) was the first day of school when she was alone for the first time. Until then, there was always a familiar face around, but her mother left her there unannounced. At that moment, she feared that her mother would never return.

Michelle's ISE took place at the age of 3 when her parents divorced. She returned home with her mother one day, and her father was gone. She recalled her mother's facial expressions and outburst of tears.

At that moment, confusion and fear set in: she felt alone, afraid and unloved. Those feelings were overwhelming. She had never felt them before, and certainly not with that intensity and not with regard to her parents.

No meaningful explanation came from her mother as Michelle tried to make sense of the event in her own Mind.

She concluded that something terrible happened, and with no reasoning voice to counter her thoughts, she believed it had something to do with herself.

This may not make sense to the adult reader, but for the child the world revolves around them. It is natural for every child at this age to assume themselves to be the cause of any effect.

Michelle's thought process was: "Before I was born, they were happy (her parents said that love brought her to them), and now they are not, therefore, it is my fault." This led her to conclude that: "If I were better or not born at all, my parents would still be happy."

Michelle's ISE revealed a moment in time when her world turned upside down. The emotional nature of that moment impressed her Mind with immense negativity: the door to her Subconscious Mind swung open, and the negative perception of self was formed.

Negative perceptions generate powerful emotions. Unexpressed or not exhausted, these emotions get "trapped inside" within our time line. Emotions, like water, need to flow: otherwise they become stale and toxic.

During the first Step of Immersive Healing, each SSE and ISE needs to be *properly identified and addressed*. The outcome of the whole process depends greatly on our ability to successfully resolve each part. The Subconscious Mind can excite feelings and emotions buried in each SSE and the ISE which allows the client to reexamine their validity in real time.

When the ISE is relived, these toxic and often intense emotions rise to the surface Emotions buried in an ISE have been brewing for many years. Our main concern is their proper and safe release. This emotional release in the Immersive Healing process is shown in Figure 16

In Michelle's case, the intense fear she felt at that moment was in direct response to her mother's emotional response and lack of communication. She knew something was very wrong, and realized there and then that her existence was not enough to prevent her mother from feeling this pain. Michelle learned for the first time that her mother's world did not revolve around her.

This is a powerful discovery for a child. It alters the child's comprehension of the world. Although no intentional harm was intended, harm was in fact done. In that respect, Michelle's mother is the "offender," and Michelle is the offended.

Often there is some sort of "unspoken" contract with the offender that prevented us from fully expressing our true feelings. Due to the "silent and unacknowledged" contract, many people find it very difficult to face their offender and express their feelings.

My preferred release method is to help my clients create (in their Mind's eye) a safe environment to properly express and exhaust their feelings and emotions. The offender can be sitting in a chair in front of them. They are unable to move, speak or even blink without their offender's specific permission. As if frozen in time, the offender must bear witness to the pain their actions inflicted and the consequences in the client's life.

For many clients, this is the first opportunity to confront the offending person, and therefore it is an emotionally charged moment. This intense energy must be released, and the client gets to do it safely by pounding repeatedly into a soft pillow while speaking their Mind freely and honestly until drained and at peace again.

After all the emotional intensity was released and the mental fog had cleared, Michelle could finally see the ISE in a broader context. This helped her realize the ISE's correct meaning, in contrast to her previously perceived incorrect meaning. She could now consider the quality of her parents' relationship (at that time) and the various individual challenges they both faced in their lives. The effect of changing perception and seeing things in their true perspective is included in Figure 16.

Michelle recognized that her parents made choices of their own. They alone were responsible for those choices. She further realized her parents' choices were made without any input from her! They chose to date, get married, have a child, and then divorce. She made none of these choices in any way, shape or form. Finally, she saw the truth hidden behind the veil of her erroneous perception of that event. Truly she was not responsible for their pain or the breakup and all that followed.

Michelle discovered that she was not the cause of their pain, but that she was its remedy. She represented the good and the pure in their relationship, the one part that worked in their lives. Accepting this truth freed her from the prison of self-hate, shame, and blame. She was ready to forgive herself.

A well known proverb says: "around every dark cloud, *there is a silver lining.*" In every bad situation there is an element of good. We can gain a benefit from every terrible thing that happens to us, and we can find meaning and purpose in each difficult or seemingly negative situation.

What was the "silver lining" in Michelle's experience? The emotional impact of the ISE on her life was immense. It forced her to develop mental and psychological mechanisms for the purpose of self-preservation.

I use the word *"forced"* because her parents' divorce was *not her choice* or her wish. Instead, she was *thrown into the water* and forced to learn how to swim in order to survive.

People who survive extremely difficult situations invariably claim to have learned something precious from their experience. In their darkest hour, they discovered aspects within, beyond words or explanation. Aspects such as inner strength, increased wisdom, and greater awareness, which helped them conduct their lives more successfully.

Michelle could begin to see a positive outcome from her difficult ordeal. Her ISE forced her to develop inner resources and mechanisms to meet life's challenges in a productive manner. Since these energies, resources and mechanisms are no longer needed to uphold her internal conflicts, they can now be used to help achieve and accomplish her desires in the world.

Her new-found understanding transformed her life. She could finally see herself in a positive light with greater self-acceptance and self-esteem, free from the crippling patterns of self-judgment and self-punishment. Her outlook changed dramatically for the better. She had more energy and felt alive for the first time in years.

Often the aftertaste of *erroneous perceptions* is guilt. Guilt arises from the many years of self-blaming and tormenting ourselves for something we did not do.

Now Michelle could see clearly how her erroneous perceptions and beliefs had influenced every aspect of her life. The doom and gloom nature of these perceptions clouded her intimate relationships, her self-worth and willingness to pursue her dreams. She needed to grieve and forgive for the years lost to these incorrect perceptions. It was time to forgive and heal herself (Figure 16) for having perceived events this way in the first place.

In Immersive Healing, forgiveness is facilitated through a series of steps or processes that incorporate forms of emotional expressions and release anchored in breathing and visualization. The result is a renewed perception of self, worthy of love, health and healing. There is a restored sense of wholeness and state of inner equilibrium.

Michelle has successfully identified and healed the ISE that her Subconscious Mind had linked to her condition. In

Regression Therapy healing takes place in the *past,* and that means her point of awareness and self-perception is still *reliving the past.* It is time to bring forth and assimilate all the *past* healing into the *present* time perception.

The process for each client is unique, and there are different ways to accomplish this goal. For Michelle, when given the suggestion to do so her Subconscious Mind regressed back to a time before her ISE occurred. She regressed back to a time when her self-perception was still intact and whole. This was a time when negativity was not yet impressed upon her, a time when she did not yet believe it was important to her. With negativity not yet in place, new perceptions with positive information and reinforcement were received, meeting no resistance from the Critical Faculty of the Conscious Mind.

Michelle showered the little girl she once was, her inner child, with love, acceptance, respect and courage. This became her identity and a prism through which she now perceives her life.

Having learned that she is allowed to feel love and is worthy of health, success and well-being, her Critical Faculty will from now on reject any information that does not reflect these qualities and attributes. A great deal of my clients session time is dedicated to this process. It assimilates our new and cleansed identity into our awareness.

At this point, Michelle's Subconscious Mind is instructed to move forward in time until it reaches the present time. Armed with a brand new mental "field of vision", the Subconscious reexamines and edits all the compounding life events within her time line, those she is aware of and those she is not, using the new perceptions to override their old perceptions, and heal them too.

It is important to understand that Immersive Healing is a systematic goal-oriented healing program with a distinct beginning, middle and end. It takes five to ten sessions to successfully complete the five steps. At the end of a session, you will leave my office intact and whole. This ensures your sense of well-being and makes it easy for you to integrate back into your daily routine.

We heal our thoughts, perceptions and beliefs. We heal our Mind and, with it, restore the conditions whereby lasting healing of the physical body can take place.

As Steve Parkhill said: "Healing is allowed to be easy, expedient, complete and permanent. The Mind's mechanisms and the universe's laws are perfectly at peace with healing."

Chapter 10

Increasing the Odds of Healing

A rift between conventional *Modern Medicine* and *Mind-Body Medicine (MBM)* has been going on for decades due to fundamental differences in their core approaches to treatment. The debate over cure versus healing of Modern Medicine and Mind-Body Medicine spans distinctions in philosophy, methodology and implementation. Modern Medicine focuses on the treatment of physical symptoms, whereas Mind-Body Medicine has adopted a more holistic approach which focuses on all dimensions that comprise the Whole Person.

Immersive Healing provides the benefits of a therapeutic process grounded in scientific research *and* a holistic approach to the patient's quality of life as its first priority.

At last patients can truly benefit from an integrated approach to healing where the skill of medical practitioners serves the physical dimension, and the skill of holistic practitioners serve all dimensions of the patient. Immersive Healing helps my clients heal the internal non-physical aspects of their illness and implement a process for a *Mind and Body* approach to healing.

Immersive Healing empowers the client to heal from within and accepts their needs, concerns, fears and hopes. Cancer patients are much more than just a failing body. The New Cancer Paradigm recognizes and respects a person's multi-dimensional nature, and therefore increases the effectiveness of medical treatment and improves the odds for healing. It recognizes not only the disease, but also the patient and their illness.

The Spectrum of Healing Practices

The fundamental distinctions between medical and non-medical practices fuel a competition between the two camps. The debate about whether one practice is better or more important than the other has no winner, certainly not the patient. It focuses on what sets the two apart, rather than on what each practice contributes to the solution.

By highlighting the advantages of each practice and how to properly integrate them, many more cancer patients will benefit. If we developed a ranking system for each practice, then the medical practice should clearly be first due to the nature, type and conditions it treats. Any threat to life or physical wound should be treated immediately without any hesitation.

However, no surgical knife, no amount of chemotherapy or psychotherapy can heal the *"Wounded" Mind*, the Subconscious Illness Paradigm. Without question, the first priority for the patient is to get illness and its symptoms under control. Nevertheless, treating only the symptom is but one part of the healing equation and definitely not the whole equation.

After the condition stabilizes, we must then strive to discover and understand what our Mind is telling us. As the body heals, it is vital and critical that we also heal emotionally and mentally.

Our multi-dimensional nature suggests that illness will occur when one-dimension is out of harmony or out of balance. Therefore, by caring for ourselves on all levels - spiritual, physical and mental - we maintain a state of health (Figure 17). The strongest position in the triangle is right in the very center. That center graphically represents the optimal position for harmony among all three dimensions.

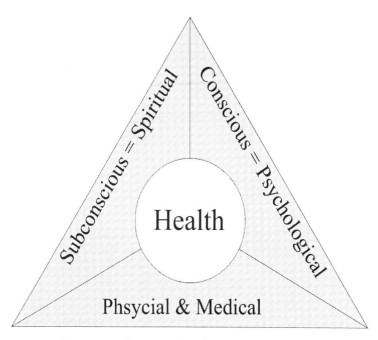

Figure 17 - The Triangle of Immersive Healing

Surgery, chemotherapy and radiation may remove the cancer cells, yet the Subconscious that calls for the illness will continue to echo through your body until it is healed. By focusing only on the physical symptoms we are but *managing our disease.* Denying our multi-dimensional nature, we fail to treat the Whole Person, and thus allow the illness to re-occur.

To permanently get rid of a yard full of dandelions, we must remove the roots, not just the stems or the visible parts. Failing to do so will only set you up to watch them return, grow and multiply all over the yard again. Ripping out only the visible stem or flower does not permanently get rid of the dandelion. My role is to help clients heal the "internal non-physical aspects" of their illness, thereby completing a total *Mind and Body* approach.

The Truth about Psychosomatic Illness

There is a common misconception of the term "psychosomatic". If we say someone has a "psychosomatic" illness, the usual misconception is that the condition is unreal and just a figment of the imagination.

The word "psychosomatic" includes psyche (Mind) and soma (Body). It means that the Body and Mind together form a complete integrated system comprising both components. One does not exist without the other.

If the Mind is affected then *the body is affected*, and if the body is affected *then the Mind will be affected*. Mind and Body cannot be separated when healing is required. Healing cannot be completed without healing the Mind and, therefore, virtually everything we experience has a psychosomatic dimension.

The Free Dictionary defines a psychosomatic illness as "a disorder whereby the physical symptoms are caused or exacerbated by psychological factors, such as migraine headache, lower-back pain, or irritable bowel syndrome. It is now recognized that emotional factors play a role in the development of nearly all organic illnesses and that the physical symptoms experienced by the patient are related to many interdependent factors, including psychological and cultural."

The physical manifestations of illness cannot be divorced from the patient's emotional life, unless it was the result of mechanical trauma. Each of us responds uniquely to the "stress" of illness, emotions affecting the sensitivity to trauma, irritating elements within the environment, susceptibility to infection, and the ability to recover from the effects of illness. A physical condition with contributory psychological factors is currently classified as *psychological factors affecting the medical condition.* Any physical condition can be so classified, but only the most frequent conditions are: asthma, peptic ulcer, bowel disorders, cardiovascular disorders, arthritis, headache and certain endocrine disorders.

The truth is that psychosomatic illness is very real and can most definitely be experienced. Because an organic origin cannot be found, it is presumed that psychological factors, emotional patterns and certain states of Mind must be responsible for the *appearance* of the physical illness.

Author Marilyn Hunter says: "It is impossible for us to be sick or injured and not have an emotional response to that, it is also impossible to be emotionally distressed *or* overjoyed and the body not respond to it." In this sense, because Mind and Body are inter-connected, all illness is psychosomatic. Every physical aspect can be traced back to the Mind. Studying the Mind aspects that influenced the body into illness may enable us to alleviate internal stress, revive the innate Immune-Response and speed up the healing process from within.

When evaluating the psychosomatic origin of illness such as cancer, we must open our minds to the possibility that certain Mind aspects played a role in influencing this condition.

Mind aspects agitated and stressed the body's internal environment over many years, disrupted its proper functioning and produced the conditions whereby the illness can thrive. Cancer can more easily develop when the Immune System is compromised.

Over the last few decades, modern Medicine's increased interest in better understanding the potent

146

relationship between the Mind and Body has given birth to the field of Psychosomatic Medicine.

Mosby's Medical Dictionary defines Psychosomatic Medicine as "a branch of Medicine concerned with the interrelationships between mental and emotional reactions and somatic processes, in particular, the manner that intra-psychic conflicts (a conflict that is a direct result of a behavior that does not justify one's beliefs) influence physical symptoms." This broader view of illness is a very promising step in the right direction.

The question is no longer "if" the Mind has a direct role in our state of health, but rather "how can we discover and harness this capacity of the Mind to reverse the process of illness and heal the body from cancer?"

With every new discovery in Psychosomatic Medicine, we increase the patient's odds of recovery. By treating the Whole Person we increase the patient's potential success rate to heal. You can beat the statistics.

Scientist Versus Healer: Divided We Fall

In my ideal world, Healer and Scientist work together. However, Healer and Scientist currently describe two practices that are far apart.

In this world, practitioners of all types recognize the value of treating both the Mind and the body, to provide patients with an integrated, comprehensive approach that will benefit them the most.

This approach acknowledges the patient's multi-dimensional nature and will greatly benefit from a multi-disciplinary treatment plan. Such a plan will ensure both a higher rate of success in treatment outcome while providing a higher quality of life during the treatment.

Would you prefer a healing plan where invasive intervention is the last resort and not the first or only treatment option? If your answer is yes, then consider a plan where your doctor prescribes therapies such as Hypnotherapy as part of your preparation regimen for surgery, radiation or chemotherapy.

A survey conducted by the National Center for Complementary Medicine found that approximately 38 percent of U.S. adults (over 18) and approximately 12 percent of the children have used some form of complementary or alternative Medicine.

One of the few things we can be sure of is that "one size fits all" Medicine does not work. Each individual patient has a unique set of circumstances that must be addressed on a one on one basis. To meet this challenge Medicine, a Personalized Medicine approach is needed whereby health care is tailored to patient's particular needs. Personalized Medicine is a medical model whereby all decisions and practices are tailored to the individual patient's genetics or other related information.

While Personalized Medicine is far superior to the existing medical practice, it is still a limiting approach because it excludes non-medical practices, and fails to address the psychosomatic nature of illness.

Failing to include the Mind in the equation of healing means failing to address the Whole Person and to heal the Whole Person.

The Placebo Effect at Work

"If any pill has been shown undeniably to work in clinical trials, it is the sugar pill common in the placebo treatment "(TIME magazine OCT.2009).

A phenomenon commonly referred to as the placebo effect is a simulated medical intervention in the form of inert tablets or sugar pills. In many cases, patients given a placebo have a perceived improvement or experience an actual improvement of a medical condition.

The word 'placebo', Latin for "I will please," was first used in a medicinal context in the 18th century. It relates to a patient's perception and positive expectation of treatment. If the substance they received was viewed as helpful, it often healed, but if it was viewed as harmful, it could cause negative effects. The negative effect is known as the 'Nocebo' effect.

The placebo has a negative connotation associated with deception or false Medicine. To a scientist, this is the truth, the whole truth: there is no active ingredient of therapeutic value in the pill or treatment, so therefore it is false.

Some clinicians go so far as considering hypnosis to be a form of placebo, but research validated that hypnotic suggestions indeed produce a very real therapeutic effect and, therefore, require no deception in order to be effective. For years, scientists dismissed the placebo effect as a figment of people's imagination and were told it was all in their head. Recently, however, researchers began using PET scanners and MRIs to examine the effect of sugar pills on the patient's brain. They discovered that the placebo effect or belief in treatment actually results in changes in brain chemistry, and is therefore very real!

Placebos are given as control treatments in medical research studies and depend on the use of measured deception. The patient receives an inert pill along with the suggestion that it may improve their condition, but is not told that the pill is inert. Just as Mr. Wright, received an injection of what he thought was a cure for cancer, but it was only pure water.

Doctors and researchers that use such interventions increase patient's belief in the treatment, and this belief produces a subjective perception of a therapeutic effect causing the patient to feel their condition has improved.

The medical community does not agree about the importance and validation of the placebo in a clinical setting. Some researchers endorse it, and some dismiss it. Some clinical trials have concluded there is no evidence, while others have revealed compelling evidence of clinical importance.

Future studies will undoubtedly continue to deepen our understanding about where, when and how placebo and Nocebo act.

In the meantime, as a non-medical practitioner, my attention is solely on the fact that some people heal their symptoms and illnesses by the sheer power of their belief in treatment. The placebo effect points to the importance of perception and the brain's role in physical health. From my perspective, this is the most interesting fact emerging from these studies. By all means, we may not yet understand why some people are able to reverse their cancer and heal their body.

Whether we call this phenomenon a placebo, the power of belief, faith healing or mental healing or any other name that excites the imagination, the bottom line is that we each have within us the capacity and resources to heal.

If one human being can heal in this way, then *we can all heal in this way*. Healing is not a privilege given to one and withheld from another. The questions researchers and scientists should be asking is: "By what means, ways, methods or mechanisms can we harness this innate healing capacity?"

Placebos do not work for everyone, but not everyone responds to an active drug either. The percentage of patients that reported relief following a placebo (39%) is comparable to the percentages following 4 mg (36%) and 6 mg (50%) of hidden morphine. (Spiegel)

One of the proposed reasons for not studying the internal mechanisms that activate the placebo for healing is based on money. Dr. Bruce Lipton, an authority on the placebo, acknowledges in his book *The Biology of Belief* that research is often funded and greatly influenced by the pharmaceutical industry.

Lipton further claims involvement by pharmaceutical companies "keeps us from looking at healing that does not involve chemicals and drugs only for the simple reason that a pharmaceutical company makes money by selling chemicals. The talk of healing yourself by using your Mind, That message does not sell very well with their corporate mission to generate profits for shareholders. It is not in the interest of the pharmaceutical industry to support "free energy" healing. It is a subject that gets no coverage except for 15 minutes about the "placebo" and then it disappears from the media radar and out of the system, and yet it is the most important new understanding (though it is not new)."

Previously, we lacked a rational explanation of how working through the Mind might be able to affect change physical or organic disease. The study of PNI, however, provides a logical explanation. In doing so PNI invites us to change the way we perceive Medicine.

Instead of depending only on external resources, now we can begin to use our own natural and innate healing capacity, and be the healers in our own lives.

Your Expectations Can Heal You

Diagnosis of a life-threatening illness is often accompanied by the negative expectancy of *a poor quality of life or even death.* Most medical practitioners follow an honest approach when talking to patients or family members when the *worst-case scenario is considered.* After all, some of those battling cancer will not survive.

It is challenging to *"sell" positive expectancy* because it is hard to measure. We can never be sure that someone with a chronic condition *really believes they have the ability to heal,* and this "belief factor" is crucial to the outcome. Mind-Body healing states that one must believe enough either in their *own ability* to heal or in *the ability* of a procedure to heal in order to experience healing.

If the client really believes healing is attainable, they are much more likely to heal. The chances of healing are greatly improved with meaningful positive belief that healing will take place. However, if they only say they believe, then the hollow words are without power. Just saying they believe in order to comfort loved ones and other then it will not work. The belief factor that creates change must be real.

Positive belief statements like *"I'm going to beat this," "I'm going to fight this thing"* need verbalization, but they must also be really and truly felt. Only when thoughts are fused with emotions can they enter the Subconscious and become a part of your new health Paradigm. The scientific validation of PNI highlights the power of our psyche, the quality of mood, the state of Mind and the expectations that affect illness and health. PNI makes it very clear that *our state of Mind and mental expectancy can either inhibit or boost Immune function.*

To employ the insight of PNI, we must change our beliefs, attitudes and expectations about healing and take ownership of our Mind. In this way we align ourselves with and harness the power of the Mind to promote health and well-being. *Thoughts do create reality only when they are transformed into intelligent and persistent action.*

All of this must be done responsibly. If you are undergoing medical treatment, follow your doctor's advice and guidelines. If you are coping with adverse treatment side-effects, give yourself time and rest.

Chapter 11

From a Victim to a Warrior

In the context of a life-threatening illness such as cancer, to be courageous means to accept illness as an experience that has both a purpose and meaning.

Courage is *the quality of Mind and/or spirit that enables a person to face difficulty, challenges, danger, pain, etc., without fear.*

Contrary to what some may think, illness is not a cruel form of heavenly punishment or bad luck, and it is not caused by evil external forces. Thinking in this way only leaves us powerless and serves no purpose. We can find no inspiration in these beliefs. To be courageous is to discover the purpose and meaning of illness, even when it means we must look inside ourselves for the answers. The journey back to good health is a great awakening and provides a deeper understanding of our relationship to life.

For many of my clients, such a moment of awakening happens when they come to realize that the *only way out is by going in*. One must shed the old non-authentic-self and reclaim life. There is tremendous transformative power in this realization, and watching them rise from the ashes of fear as warriors is invaluable.

We have a choice of how to respond when we meet face to face with cancer. In the words of Shawna Myrick, the mother of three-year-old Liam Myrick who is struggling with Neuroblastoma, *"you either get bitter, or you get better."*

I believe we cannot *control the cause of cancer*, but we *can influence its course*. It takes tremendous courage, determination, and strength to cultivate and keep a fighting spirit in the face of so many challenges, *but it is possible*. Strengthen your inner warrior by reminding yourself that you have value and worth extending beyond your current physical condition. Above all, remind yourself that while your journey is unique, you are not alone.

Coping with the Shock of Cancer Diagnosis

Each healing journey starts with bad news. A cancer diagnosis challenges even the most optimistic Mind and forces us to *"think the unthinkable"*.

We fear cancer more than any other illness because at one time the word cancer conveyed a death sentence. This is outdated thinking because more and more people survive their cancer today than at any other time in medical history. Nevertheless, the nature of bad news itself is debilitating. Many of my clients described the moment they were first diagnosed as a defining moment in their life, and afterwards nothing stayed the same.

We take the first step toward healing when we acknowledge and face our fear. Unpleasant as it may be, this will help us to shorten the *wait-and-recovery* time between receiving the bad news and the healing process.

Facing our fear also means a faster transition between feeling like a victim and setting forth on the empowered path of the warrior. *The sooner we face the fear, the quicker we move from victim to warrior and fight the battle.*

The stakes are high and the vicious *cycle of fearful thoughts* puts us at risk of falling into the common *Mind traps of hopelessness and helplessness.* Research shows hopelessness and helplessness have a negative impact on our health.

Our priority is to pay particular attention to our feelings. Respect and express your feelings so as to avoid the Mind traps and remain hopeful and determined to heal.

Ignoring our feelings, or not acknowledging or expressing what we feel inside, does not make them disappear. As the saying goes, *that which we resist the most tends to persist.*

Give yourself permission to tune into your emotions: they will point you in the right direction to the place within that needs the most attention and healing.

The Courage to Heal

The first step to begin the healing process is summoning *the courage to heal.* Courage is necessary to break free from cultural, social or personal fixed beliefs about illness. Breaking free of *"body-only"* thinking takes courage. There is a great sense of ownership and recognition for those who have the audacity to stand up for their lives and survive.

Intuitively we know that both health and illness are expressions of our internal environment. We know this to be true because we only become aware or pay attention to our body when it hurts! Only when pain is present or when we become ill do we take notice of our physical body.

We fear what we might find inside and tend to put our lives on hold rather than seek professional help. Since *fear is debilitating*, we must summon the courage to overcome it and face our deepest innermost beliefs. It takes great courage to challenge our thoughts and emotions, and to take ownership of who we are.

Courage is also necessary to overcome social and individual perceptions of cancer. Unfortunately consumer literature and media focus on the number of people who lost the battle with cancer, with little mention about the survivors. It is this negative view of cancer that we must face courageously and overcome.

We can view our illness as an opportunity for change and personal growth. If embraced correctly, illness can be a turning point to a new and purposeful life.

Courage is not the absence of fear *but the acquired ability to move beyond fear.* Mr. Wright had the courage to look beyond fear. Mr. Wright's story, and others like it, demonstrate that beliefs can influence what happens on a cellular level in the body. All it takes is your courage to take responsibility and action for your life situation, to decide that you will heal, and to believe that you can influence the health of your cells.

The most prominent emotion in our modern society is fear. We are fearful or frightened of losing what we have worked for, rejection, failure, financial loss, relationships, other people, criticism, suffering, heartaches, change, and letting others know what is really on our Mind.

Often we are reluctant to be true to ourselves and allow others to see our truth. We are *consciously* aware of some of our fears while other fears *exist subconsciously*. Fear, thoughts, and emotions play a major role in directing not only our action, but also in how our physical body responds. Fear can imprison and paralyze the human spirit. *Courage sets us on the path to healing.*

"Now is the time and opportunity to stop viewing life's challenges as stumbling blocks but change them to become stepping stones." Avinoam Lerner (2012)

Fear is Just a Four Letter Word

Anyone who heard the words *"you have cancer"* knows their devastating power. Understandably the first response is fear.

Fear is often fueled by poor self-image. This is a thought process stating that we do not have the resources to cope and heal, and that we may not be worthy of healing.

We must have a proper coping mechanism in place to survive debilitating fear! Fear can color every aspect of our life with dark clouds and gloom, and give birth to hopelessness and despair.

One client said that fear made her feel as if her field of vision narrowed from wide open and bright to narrow and dark. She said it affected her as if she walked through a corridor with many different doors, each door leading to another piece of her life.

Others describe fear as feeling detached and removed, like watching a movie, while others feel overwhelmed and debilitated.

Regardless of the experience, it is clear that we need a practical, realistic and effective protocol to deal with fear and its side-effects.

Three Point Strategy for Handling Fear

1. Understand fear letter by letter. The online Free Dictionary defines this word F.E.A.R - False Evidence Appear Real.

2. See the big picture. Many people may still think of cancer as incurable, but this is simply *not* the case today. More and more people survive cancer due to advanced treatments and new technology.

3. Remember the truth about statistics. *Statistics are just numbers.* Statistics do not heal or create illness.

Every one of us is unique. We all have different DNA and a unique mental, emotional and spiritual makeup. If we were alike in every sense, there would be just one treatment, and it would work for everyone. Do not be tempted to associate yourself with specific statistics and forecast your future! Keep in Mind *all those who survived and outlived the statistics.* You will be the next one!

A True Case of Courage and Inspiration

Some people *appear to beat the odds* and have *"special powers"* that inspire others to emerge as heroes when all hope is lost. If this power *exists in all people,* then what is this *"special"* talent? A client once said to me "*bad things happen only to good people*" when referring to his stage three colon cancer. There was little I could say to convince him otherwise than to offer a quote by Dennis Wholey: "*Expecting the world to treat you fairly, because you are a good person, is a little like expecting a bull not to attack you because you are a vegetarian.*" A few days later he told me that this quotation transformed his outlook and made him realize he is far from being a victim.

This client is a hero in my eyes, a person of courage and strength. He faced what he feared the most, what caused him to feel *helpless and hopeless.* In a following session he said: "I just refuse to let my fear of dying run my life anymore. If it is my time to go, I will do so fighting for my life."

Once again, the hero emerged, strong and powerful, no longer helpless and hopeless. He chose to see his physical symptoms, fatigue and discomfort as part of the natural world. He viewed it as part of the eternal cycle of life, in all of its terrible beauty. This takes great courage.

Chapter 12

Integrating Immersive Healing in your Treatment Plan

Conventional Medicine has made great strides and breakthroughs in developing *less invasive* cancer treatments. Nowadays more people survive cancer, and that is the *positive bottom line*.

However, the fact remains that chemotherapy, radiation therapy and surgery take a very heavy toll on patients.

Invasive medical treatments, harsh side-effects, disruptions to the quality of life and daily routine *affect both the patient and their family*. Fear and uncertainty lead to feeling distraught, helpless and not being in control. It casts a shadow that suggests a state of Mind that *"I am not well."*

This is yet one more reason why Immersive Healing, which utilizes Hypnotherapy as its therapeutic vehicle, is such a powerful tool to incorporate into any conventional cancer treatment plan. Hypnotherapy helps patients cope and mobilize their inner resources for healing. Doing so restores their sense of living and being in control of their life. Immersive Healing is designed to work alongside conventional medical treatment to help achieve that goal.

Here are four key reasons I believe integrating Hypnotherapy will help you achieve that goal. These four reasons explain how this safe, non-invasive, drugless and painless practice accomplishes that goal.

Reason 1 – Enhances Medical Treatment Efficacy

The onset of cancer or any life-threatening illness is extremely taxing both emotionally and physically. Stress, fear and anxiety take over as we try to make sense of our new reality. We need something to hold on to, something that will motivate us to navigate our lives back to safety.

Researchers found that stress and hopelessness, as well as other debilitating emotions, disrupt and suppress the functioning of the Immune System. In order to revive the Immune System, we must negate these harmful states of Mind.

Hypnosis *first* allows the client to *change their perception about treatment outcome from dire to hopeful.* It can then increase belief in their ability to cope with the challenges that lay ahead. At that point, hypnosis can be used to access the Subconscious Mind - the part of the Mind governing all bodily functions, including Immune function - to identify and heal the beliefs and perceptions that caused the state of stress or hopelessness. Hypnosis is the key to Immersive Healing.

Once the conditions inhibiting the proper functioning of the Immune System have been addressed, it will return to its normal function. This in turn provides an advantage to become well once again.

A strengthened Immune System and healed Mind enable other medical treatments to work more efficiently and effectively. In other words, the patient's body will then accept medical and other types of healing more readily with less resistance.

Immersive Healing works hand in hand with other treatments to help you along the path to regaining your health.

Reason 2 – Reduces the Amount of Medical Intervention Needed

A growing body of research confirms that patients using hypnosis (Hypnotherapy) in preparation for surgery require less anesthesia and medication. Furthermore, patients using Hypnotherapy healed much faster from surgery than the control group. This is a very significant improvement. Using hypnosis before *any* surgery or other medical treatment can help decrease the worries, fears, stress and anxieties leading up to the treatment. Most of the fear comes from the feeling of *being out of control*. Fear may manifest itself as a feeling that the body is in a deteriorating state of health and that nothing can bring it to a halt. Hypnotherapy is used to address the *psychological* impact of diagnosis and treatment in this case. Entering treatment with the right frame of Mind can potentially reduce the amount of overall medical interventions or Medicine.

Dr. Guy Montgomery from Mount Sinai School of Medicine led a study of 200 women with breast cancer. His research found that patients who used hypnosis before surgery needed fewer anesthetics during surgery. They also reported less pain, nausea, fatigue and emotional distress *after surgery*. . Hospitalization was reduced by as much as nine days.

Severe side effects of breast cancer surgery can mean longer hospital stays, additional drugs, or a return to the hospital ward when the patient should be recovering at home. Properly preparing patients both mentally and psychologically can result in less time in the hospital and an easier return to normal life.

Reason 3 – Maintains a High Quality of Life

The therapeutic application of hypnosis (Hypnotherapy) helps the client to mobilize inner resources for healing.

Hypnotherapy uses our thoughts, emotions, beliefs and perceptions to influence the physical body

This makes Hypnotherapy a safe, non-invasive, drugless and painless natural practice. As such, Hypnotherapy requires no hospital stay and no medication, so our sense of well-being and quality of life remains high.

Hypnotherapy uses the power of the spoken word, statements, and suggestions to produce a therapeutic effect in the body. In that respect, Hypnotherapy as outlined in Immersive Healing can be thought of as a *Mind Operation* one that leaves no scars and is very safe. Unlike medical operations, it requires no sedation and the client remains in control at all times.

Numerous studies have explored the efficacy of hypnosis in enhancing patients' quality of life (Liossi and White 2001) (Laidlaw and Willett 2002) (Laidlaw, Bennett, Dwivedi, Naito and Gruzelier 2005). The results were promising. In all these studies, patients in the hypnosis group reported significantly better quality of life and lower levels of anxiety and depression, as compared to the standard care group.

Reason 4 – Healing in All Dimensions

Illness is usually accompanied by an uneasy feeling or sense that *something is not 'right' within the body*. Something has caused *an imbalance*. However we *have not learned where to find the imbalance* or how to correct it so that health can be restored.

From the perspective of a healer, illness is *more* than just a physical event. The body and the Mind are an integrated system, and change in one part causes change in the other. If the physical body is affected, it is very likely that some factors or aspects of the Mind are involved. By healing the "Mind" aspects, we can support the body and reinstate health.

Hypnotherapy enables the search for these factors and aspects, and therefore shines brighter than any other healing modality. Hypnotherapy allows us to *look deeper into the meaning of our condition* and allows us *hear the silent cry of our Subconscious Mind.*

It is no coincidence that we experience a change in our state of health after periods of intense stress or worry.

Feeling sick or like we might be coming down with something forces us to slow down and rest. Though we may not be aware, the Subconscious is telling us to pay attention and take better care of our health.

The body broadcasts a cry of illness with symptoms telling you that something is not working properly and that you should take some corrective action. Immersive Healing allows you to identify, resolve and heal the Subconscious 'stressors' or Subconscious Illness Paradigm that promoted the conditions that led to the illness.

Healing the Subconscious Illness Paradigm means allowing the body to ignite and revive its natural Immune-Response. It means strengthening *your will-to-live*, a very significant and important aspect in the healing process.

The truth remains: *"Changes made in the Mind bring about changes in the body."* Changes may include; an enhanced and properly functioning Immune System and a level of physical comfort which helps you to follow through and complete your medical treatment.

Immersive Healing can harnesses the innate healing ability of the Mind. Integrating Immersive Healing and Hypnotherapy into your cancer treatment can help to heal the root cause of your illness.

Chapter 13

Questions and Answers about Immersive Healing

Being informed and asking questions gives you some control and may help you cope. Studies show people with cancer who are fully informed about their disease and treatment options usually tend to heal better and have fewer side-effects than those who simply follow doctors' orders. Some people feel overwhelmed by too much information, or do not want to know as many details about their condition.

Is Immersive Healing for Me?

Immersive Healing is a goal-oriented approach to healing designed to help cancer patients heal from within. If you want to be more in control of your health, to overcome fear and distress, and to increase your body's resilience, then Immersive Healing is an option you should explore.

Can Everyone Benefit from Hypnotherapy?

If you have imagination and can visualize or "see" in your Mind's eye, you can benefit from hypnosis. Anyone who is willing to follow instructions can be hypnotized.

Is hypnosis mind control?

No. You are in control throughout the session. In fact, your Mind will alert you or simply reject any suggestion that does not reflect your own desire to change. Hypnosis is a natural state of Mind that occurs when the Mind is focused, and your attention is absorbed in the process.

What if I can't get out of hypnosis?

There is *no such a thing as getting "stuck"* in hypnosis, no more than you can get stuck reading a book or watching a movie. All it takes to emerge from hypnosis is your decision to stop.

How many sessions should I plan?

Immersive Healing requires a minimum of five sessions. A typical program runs from five to ten sessions. For some clients, five sessions is plenty to reach their goal. For others, more sessions may be needed. The program structure is tailored to each client's individual needs.

Will I experience immediate results from my session?

You will certainly feel that you are on the right track and that Immersive Healing is promoting change from within. However, it is important to be realistic and remember that healing is a process that takes time. Be patient with your body and with yourself, and the benefits will follow.

Will I be able to hear and remember is said while in hypnosis?

Yes, you will hear every word either you or I have said. In addition, you will be able to remember everything about your session. Hypnosis is a state of focused attention, and as such, you will hear and be aware of words and suggestions as well as feelings and emotions.

Is hypnosis similar to sleep?

Hypnosis is a term derived from the Greek word *Hypnos* for sleep, but it is not a state of sleep. While hypnosis is a state of focused attention, sleep is more a state of unconsciousness. While in hypnosis, people are aware of their surroundings in a detached sort of way. Conscious critical thinking is more or less temporarily suspended and yet available at a moment's notice to cope with an emergency if one were to come up. Some hypnotists use the word "sleep" as a call to action meaning to *close your eyes and go deeply relaxed as if you are asleep.* More specifically to Immersive Healing, a dynamic hypnotic protocol requires your active participation.

What does it feels like to be hypnotized?

You have been hypnotized before, but you may have not have called it hypnosis, or being in a hypnotic state. Hypnosis happens naturally when we allow ourselves to become deeply absorbed in a good book or a movie, or by something intriguing or important.

From my experience, people expect to feel something special or different when in hypnosis. However, because hypnosis is a natural, common and often daily experience, it is hard for them to register it as such. For the most part, people feel very relaxed and comfortable during hypnosis with little desire to move or open their eyes, *although it is totally possible.*

Because you allow yourself to be hypnotized does not in any way imply or mean you are gullible! It simply means you have allowed your Mind to become absorbed and immersed in your experience.

While in hypnosis, you may feel physical sensations such as:

- *Numbness in your hands and legs*
- *A deep sense of comfort and relaxation*
- *A sense of lightness or heaviness*
- *Tingling sensations or pleasant shivers throughout the body*
- *Greater awareness of your feelings*

These sensations merely signify that you allow yourself to enter into a hypnotic state, and are very normal.

What type of cancer will Immersive Healing work with?

Immersive Healing can be practiced with any type of cancer. This is because Immersive Healing aims at the root cause of illness rather than its symptom, expression or label.

What lifestyle changes will I need to make during Immersive Healing?

No lifestyle changes are necessary. Your quality of life will be maintained and supported throughout your sessions.

Are there side-effects with Immersive Healing?

As a Mind-Body therapy, Immersive Healing has no negative side-effects. It is a safe, non-invasive, drugless and painless process. Because no medication is involved, there are no side-effects.

Will Immersive Healing hinder my ability to perform my usual daily activities?

No. While it is important to give yourself time to assimilate the healing, your day-to-day routine will not be disturbed.

What medical information will be needed to treat me with Immersive Healing?

Information will be needed concerning your use of psychiatric medications (may affect your perception and emotional output). Also if there are physical limitations restricting your ability to sit in a recliner for a long time.

Is there anything I need to do to prepare myself for Immersive Healing?

No. The only prerequisite to Immersive Healing is your decision to heal and willingness to be guided through this process.

Do you need information about me before you treat me with Immersive Healing?

No. To determine if Immersive Healing is right for you, a short consultation will be scheduled.

Is there any information I need to share with my friends and loved ones?

This is completely up to you. Some people feel empowered by sharing their experiences, while others see their healing as an intimate experience too personal to share.

Can a friend or family member attend Immersive Healing sessions with me?

They are welcome to come with you to your initial consultation, but not to sit through your sessions. The presence of another person in your sessions inhibits honest expression of feelings and emotions, making it counterproductive to your healing.

Does it make any difference in the type or location of my cancer?

No. Immersive Healing is not concerned with the type or location but rather its root cause, i.e., the Mind patterns that created it.

Should I use Immersive Healing along with my other treatments?

Yes. Immersive Healing can be practiced in conjunction with conventional medical treatment to improve your treatment efficacy, or prior to medical treatment where it can work to lessen the amount of treatment needed.

What is the goal of the Immersive Healing?

The primary goal of Immersive Healing is to heal the Subconscious patterns and factors believed to have produced the internal conditions for illness to thrive. Its secondary goal is reviving and strengthening the natural defense system of the body, i.e., the Immune System.

Who will be part of the Immersive Healing team?

You and I work together as a team. We walk this journey together, side by side and shoulder to shoulder to ensure a successful process from beginning to end.

What is the expected timeline for my Immersive Healing Treatment?

The timeline is five to ten sessions, ideally once a week. If time is of the essence, sessions can be scheduled more frequently.

What are the short-term benefits of Immersive Healing?

Short-term benefits may include hopeful feelings and a stronger will-to-live.

What long-term benefits are associated with Immersive Healing?

Some of the long-term benefits include self-acceptance, a positive outlook on life, enhanced Immune function and ultimately healing.

Will Immersive Healing affect my fertility (ability to become pregnant or father children)?

No, it will not. In fact, by resolving the mental patterns inhibiting the proper functioning of the body, Immersive Healing may increase your fertility.

Can Immersive Healing be used with children, teenagers, young adults, and older adults?

Immersive Healing can be useful to both adults as well as teenagers. Hypnosis is not appropriate for children under 10. Personally, I work only with adults over the age of 21. I have found that working with children usually means working with their parents. This presents a completely new dynamic that impairs my ability to practice.

What follow-up will I need after Immersive Healing sessions, and how often will I need them?

Life after treatment as a cancer survivor can be challenging, both physically and emotionally. It takes time to recover and transition back to your regular life.

Three follow-up sessions are scheduled once a month to support you during this period. In this way, long-term progress can be assessed, supplemented and maintained.

Chapter 14

In-Home Exercises

Four Basic Steps to Develop Resilience

Resilience means "the positive capacity to cope with stress and adversity." Developing the skill of resilience takes time and practice. You should try the following shortcuts:

1. Accept Change: Change is a part of life. This change should be viewed as an opportunity to grow in new directions. Letting go of what cannot be changed helps you focus on what you can actually do.
2. Action Plan: Craft an action plan to negate your stress. Taking care of you is your number one priority. Do what you enjoy most: feed your body, relax your Mind and get plenty of rest.
3. Positive View: Nurture a positive view of yourself. Prime your Body and Mind with positive self-talk, be kind and supportive of you, trust that you have appropriate resources to cope, and remember that you are much more than just your body.
4. Set healthy personal boundaries. When you need space, ask for it. Those who love you may not know how to demonstrate their love and affection for you. They do not know what treatment feels like and what it is like to be you. Help them by letting them know what is right for you.

Illness, Health and your Authentic-Self

From a spiritual perspective, disease is the ultimate act of separation from the source of life and well-being. In this sense, restoring this connection will lead to restoring the body's state of health.

This is easier to say than to do because most people have little or no awareness of the part that is whole and healed, let alone the knowledge of *how* to go about restoring the connection to its source.

A valuable clue comes in the form of the following quote by Sarah Ban Breathnach: "The authentic-self is the soul made visible." These words reveal the character of that part within that is healed and whole and suggests the authentic-self as the bridge between the spirit (intangible) and our experience (tangible).

We can view the authentic-self as the sum of our values, beliefs and perceptions,

Our inner compass and inner guidance system makes it possible for us to stay true to who we are as we travel the road during life's challenges.

People who remain true to their core inner values and live in alignment with their moral codes tend to be healthier. Those able to maintain that alignment seem happier, less concerned with the harsh aspects of reality or other external stressors, and therefore less vulnerable or less affected by them emotionally, mentally and physically.

However, what does it mean to be authentic or live authentically? Children are by nature completely authentic. Though we all have started our lives this way, we changed and morphed as we grew up and met social and family dynamics head on. As adults we are usually accustomed to wearing different masks and costumes. Some serve us well while many not. This makes it hard to remember what it felt like being truly authentic.

Nevertheless, rediscovering and reconnecting with our authentic self is certainly worth the effort. The benefits are many, especially from the perspective of health and well-being.

The following three simple steps are your action plan, your strategy to rediscovering and reconnecting with your authentic self.

Step 1: Identify your core values and evaluate what changes you need to make in order to fit them in your life. For example, if one of your core values is honesty, communicating with those around you in an honest way will make you feel better and increase your self-esteem.

Step 2: Bring to Mind some of your childhood dreams, goals or people who have inspired you. Write them down and evaluate them based on those that make you feel the most excited, happiest or inspired.

Step 3: Consider what is standing in your way to accomplishing these goals and dreams, what will it take you to grow as a person in a certain way.

The bottom line is you can take steps to achieve, accomplish and become all that you know you can be. This is the path to living life more authentically and living your personal truth.

Three Stress Management Tools

The negative impact of stress on our lives is pervasive. The more we can manage our Mind the more we can help and support our body.

The foundation of stress management is a balanced Mind and a healthy lifestyle. Using the following strategies, you too can enjoy a calmer Mind and Body.

1. Interrupt your Mind.

If your body tenses up and emotions rise to the surface, take a long deep breath. A deep breath forces the Mind to focus on physical sensations, thus interrupting the aggravating thought process that cause you to feel stressed.

2. Express yourself in the right time and place.

This option might be in your best interest if the situation fits. Share your feelings with those who value and love you. Thoughts are scarier in the realm of the Mind, so put them down on paper or find another creative way to express the way you feel. *"That which we resist the most persists."*

3. Release and let go

Generally we say and do things to ourselves that we would not allow anyone else to do. In that respect we may intentionally or unintentionally blame ourselves for our illness. The pattern of self-blame and guilt breed even more emotional suffering and negatively influence our health.

We Are Not Responsible for Our Illness!

Illness is not the result of a faulty personality or lack of a good mental attitude. It is the product of many years of conditioning, believing, perceiving, etc. These processes took place below our conscious awareness in the Subconscious Mind. We are not responsible for it in any way. If illness was the result of a certain conscious mental attitude, then we could easily remove it and make it go away. If you are holding yourself responsible for your illness, it is time to release that belief. Understand that you have done the best with what you knew at that time.

As Maya Angelo said *"Now that you know better you can do better."*

List of Figures and Illustrations:

Table of Abbreviations:

AMA	American Medical Association
DMP	Disharmonious Mind Patterns
FDA	Food and Drug Administration
IH	Immersive Healing
ISE	Initial Sensitizing Event
MBM	Mind-Body Medicine
RTC	Regression to Cause
SIP	Subconscious Illness Paradigm
SSE	Subsequent Sensitizing Event
SCM	Subconscious Mind
SCMP	Subconscious Mind Paradigm

Credits & Bibliography

American Cancer Society, Inc. ©2010

Barrios, Dr. Alfred, Breaking Free with SPC (NXTGEN-2012), Towards Greater Freedom and Happiness

Choron, 1963, Grof and Halifax, 1978)

Berland, 1994, Hawley, 1989, Hirshberg and Barasch, 1995,

Huebscher, 1992, Roud, 1985)

Hannel, Charles F., The Master Key System (1912)

Hay Louise, Heal *Your Body* Klopfer, Psychologist Dr.Klopfer

Kein Gerald F, Omni Hypnosis Center in Florida, The Human Mind Model

Nietzsche, Friedrich, Twilight of the Idols (1888)

Lipton, Dr.Bruce, The Biology of Belief, Hay House Inc., (2005)

Parkhill, Stephen *Answer Cancer – the Healing of a Nation*

Ritberger Carol, PhD, Healing Happens with Your Help 2008

Rubin, Jason M., "Therapist uses hypnosis as weapon," Jewish Advocate (2012, Special to the Advocate)

Planck Dr. Max, Nobel Prize in Physics

Viktor, Frankl, M.D., Ph.D. Professor of Neurology and Psychiatry at the University of Vienna Medical School, Will to Meaning. 1969

Index

A

American Cancer Society, *21, 118, 190*
American Medical Association (AMA), *20*
Anger, *131*
Answer Cancer – The Healing of a Nation, *78*
authenticity, *103, 105, 107, 108, 111, 135*
Authenticity, *105, 106, 107, 111*

B

biotherapy, *22, 97*
Biotherapy, *23*

C

call for self-mutilation, *33*
cancer treatment, *19, 24, 31, 41, 95, 99, 121, 168, 172*
Carol Ritberger, Ph.D, *45*
Change an incorrect perception, *120*
chemotherapy, *22, 23, 24, 30, 31, 97, 101, 114, 115, 151, 168*
Chemotherapy, *22, 80, 99, 114, 117*
Clean the ISE, *120*
Conditioning Process, *64, 65, 66, 67, 68, 69, 93, 188*
Conscious Mind, *49, 50, 53, 54, 56, 90, 103, 106, 121, 136*
Conventional Medicine, *62, 168*
courage, *14, 15, 47, 131, 148, 162, 164, 165, 167*
Courage, *162, 164, 165, 167*
Critical Faculty, *76, 84, 106, 121, 122, 136, 148*

D

Dave Elman, *101*
deep-seated patterns of cancer, *30*
Dimensional Ontology, *38, 41, 47, 80, 103, 188*
Disharmonious Mind Patterns, *74*
Dr. Ader, *96*
Dr. Al Barrios, *10, 95*
Dr. Bernie Siegel, *20*
Dr. Bruce Lipton, *48, 159*
Dr. David Felten, *94*
Dr. Klopfer, *35*
Dr. Lipton, *49*
Dr. Michael Schmitz, *117*
Dr. Philip West, *18*
Dr.Klopfer, *25, 190*
Drs. Kiecolt-Glase, *95*
Dual Mind, *50*

E

emotions, 36, 38, 45, 48, 61, 62, 70, 71, 72, 77, 78, 85, 93, 95, 103, 107, 108, 110, 120, 131, 137, 140, 154, 160, 164, 165, 170, 174, 178, 185
Episodic Memory, *112*
erroneous and harmful perceptions, *108*
erroneous perception, 110, 122, 136, 143
erroneous perceptions, *45, 71, 78, 92, 107, 122, 146*

ISBN 978-1480079939

ISBN 1480079936

LCCN: 2012919144

Copyright 2012 Avinoam Lerner

USA: 24.95
Canada: 27.95

avinoamlerner.com

Blum Resource Center
Dana-Farber
450 Brookline Ave., Y-143
Boston, MA 02215
617-632-3751

GAYLORD FG

15768236R00099